Paleo
from
a to Z

Paleo
from
a to Z

A reference guide to **better health** through nutrition and lifestyle
How to eat, live and thrive as nature intended!

DARRYL EDWARDS

EXPLORER
Publishing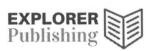

Disclaimer: This book conveys the author's opinions and ideas
based on his research as well as each of his experiences with his
clients. It has been written and published strictly for informational,
and educational purposes only and in no way should be used as a
substitute for consultation with health care professionals. The author
is providing you with the information in this work so that you can
have the knowledge and can choose, at your risk, to act on that
knowledge. The author urges all readers to be aware of their health
status and to consult medical professionals before beginning any
health, diet or lifestyle programme.

ENDORSEMENTS

"If you are looking for a simple way to better understand Paleo concepts, Darryl's *Paleo from A to Z* guide is the go-to resource."
—**Mark Sisson**, best-selling author of *The Primal Blueprint* and publisher of Mark's Daily Apple

"Don't you wish you had a translator to help you sift through the jargon and explain it all in easy-to-understand English so you can become empowered to make better health choices? Well look no further than Darryl Edwards' book *Paleo from A to Z*. This book is a micro encyclopacdia of key terms for all things Paleo. You'll find yourself returning to this unique reference, time and time again."
—**Jimmy Moore**, health blogger, podcaster, and author of *Keto Clarity* and *Cholesterol Clarity*

"Another excellent resource to get you started on your health and healing journey!"
—**Terry Wahls, M.D.**, best-selling author of *The Wahls Protocol*

"Darryl has put together what is sure to be the go-to reference for all things Paleo. This, fun, easy-to-navigate guide covers everything and anything Paleo related and will be an indispensable resource for anyone looking to lead a healthier lifestyle."
—**Cain Credicott**, founder/editor in chief of *Paleo Magazine*

ALSO BY DARRYL EDWARDS
Paleo Fitness: *Primal Training and Nutrition to Get Lean, Strong and Healthy*

Dedicated to Ne: 7/7

CONTENTS

PREFACE

"THE DEVIATION OF MAN FROM THE STATE IN WHICH HE WAS ORIGINALLY PLACED BY NATURE SEEMS TO HAVE PROVED TO HIM A PROLIFIC SOURCE OF DISEASES."

—EDWARD JENNER

In today's technology-driven, internet-enabled, health-conscious world we are more informed about our bodies than at any other time in human history and are fortunate to live in this golden age of information. We are obsessed with living longer, happier, and healthier lives. However, there's a catch. We have arguably accomplished only a third of that goal—living longer—but can we honestly say we have access to the happier and healthier parts of the equation?

Heart disease is the number one killer globally, responsible for 30 per cent of all deaths. Millions are advised to take statins to lower cholesterol and prevent heart attacks. These are some of the best-selling medicines in history, producing billions of dollars in sales. However, research suggests that even though statins are efficacious at lowering cholesterol, they only prevent heart attacks for about one in every 100 people, and there is no difference in the numbers of lives saved. The vast majority of individuals receive no health benefit from the treatment, and this does not even take into account the potential side effects, which include cognitive impairment and muscle pain. The harm-benefit equation, often tipped to the left-hand side, concerns the use of many drugs, not just statins. For example, an Australian study in March 2015 that looked at thirteen randomised, controlled studies found that paracetamol was no better than a dummy pill when it came to treating lower back pain. With the drug doing nothing to improve the sufferers' recovery time, pain levels, sleep, or quality of life. The research did highlight an association of taking paracetamol with an increase of four times the risk of liver toxicity in patients. What would work better in both examples? Lifestyle changes, such as exercise, diet, stress management, and weight reduction.

Despite all the wonders of modern medicine, the fundamental fact remains that if you are a healthy individual in today's society, you are in the minority; we are information rich, but health poor. The statistics paint an alarming picture. At the beginning of the 1900s, the majority of deaths globally were due to infectious diseases such as diarrhoea, influenza, and tuberculosis. Since the 1940s, the majority of deaths in the United States have been a result of heart disease, cancer, and other degenerative diseases, and this phenomenon has spread to the rest of the world. In 2008, the World Health Organisation (WHO) reported that 63 per cent of global deaths were due to lifestyle diseases, most of which are preventable. By 2012, that number had risen to 68 per cent.

Obesity has tripled since the 1980s, with more than a third of children in the United Kingdom being overweight or obese in 2013, and the WHO forecast that rates will continue to rise. Three in four men and two in three women in the UK will be overweight or obese by 2030, according to the UK Health Forum. In some of Europe's worst performing countries, including Ireland and Belgium, the WHO predicts that almost all adults will be overweight within fifteen years. At the same time, anorexia and bulimia are running at historically high levels.

Where have we gone wrong? On the one hand, we have diagnostic tests, cutting-edge medical treatments, highly qualified clinicians, and best-selling diet books. On the other hand, we have the backdrop of reward-seeking behaviours—labour-saving devices, binge eating, binge drinking, then before the summer vacation, binge dieting and binge exercising. Not exactly healthy. Even with health-related facts and figures at our disposal we still suffer from stressed, sleep-deprived, sedentary, socially disconnected lives. The chronic lifestyle disease epidemic shows no sign of abating any time soon, and health costs are rising faster than our ability to meet them.

It turns out that one possible solution comes from taking cues from our hunter-gatherer ancestors, a lifestyle that framed for humankind our genetic heritage: our link with past and future—eating better food, getting quality sleep, and moving our bodies as nature intended. I suspect, though, that most of you already know this and have already adopted the Paleo lifestyle or are about to begin the journey.

However we don't want to overly romanticise the past, our ancestors had many problems especially relating to low life expectancy. Carl Haub, world leading paleo-demographer at the Population Reference Bureau (PRB) claims in the Population Today report *How Many People Have Ever Lived on Earth?*, that *"life expectancy at birth probably averaged ten years for most of human history"*. His estimates suggest that 40 per cent of the human race did not survive beyond their first birthday. They suffered from diseases of microbes, many of which we have conquered. Today we suffer chronically from diseases of civilisation—most of which we can develop or avoid through lifestyle.

The goal of this book is to help you get back to basics with a handy, alphabetical reference for beginners who need some extra information. The book is also useful for those experienced with the Paleo lifestyle and want some fine tuning.

This guide presents some of the terms you will come across when reviewing information online, listening to podcasts, or having discussions with friends. It is designed to give you quick descriptions in plain English so you spend less time reading and more time living.

I urge you to eschew short-term gains and instead make following a healthy lifestyle a lifetime habit. With that in mind, I offer you *Paleo from A to Z: A Reference Guide to Better Health Through Nutrition and Lifestyle. How to Eat, Live and Thrive as Nature Intended!*

Darryl Edwards, The Fitness Explorer

PALEO FROM A TO Z

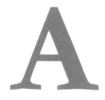

"IF WE COULD GIVE EVERY INDIVIDUAL THE
RIGHT AMOUNT OF NOURISHMENT AND
EXERCISE, NOT TOO LITTLE AND NOT TOO
MUCH, WE WOULD HAVE FOUND THE SAFEST
WAY TO HEALTH."

—HIPPOCRATES

About This Book – This book is designed to be a glossary of terms for those new to the *Paleo lifestyle* who would like a handy reference guide based on many of the questions the author has been asked over the years. It is intended to be non-intimidating and in plain English. It is not possible to answer every question you may have about Paleo, and the list is not exhaustive, but it does provide a useful starting point and will enable you to spend less time on Google searching for the very basics, assist in exploring areas of interest, and most importantly, give you more time to live a healthier lifestyle.

About This Thing Called Paleo – In the past few years, the word *Paleo* has become synonymous with a diet and lifestyle that many people have commenced to enhance their overall health, either by improving their body composition or as a way to fight and prevent disease. The Paleolithic (Palaeolithic UK) era, when stone tools were used in hunting and gathering societies, covered more than 2.5 million years and ended around 20,000 years ago. The foods of this period consisted of meat, fish, fowl, eggs, vegetables, nuts, and fruits and excluded sugar, grains, dairy, *legumes* (beans), *salt*, and processed and artificial foods.

The *Paleo diet* is a modern interpretation of what our ancestors ate as *hunter-gatherers*, a way to reduce the impact of manmade and cultivated foods introduced into the human food chain only relatively recently. Although our world has altered radically in the last 10,000 years, the human genome has hardly changed since then. One key driving theory behind the Paleo diet is that modern human's digestive systems are not designed to handle the refined sugars, grains, legumes, and dairy products that are now commonplace in the Western diet.

Acid/Alkaline Balance – A key concept from the alkaline diet that concludes that when the body's level of acid is too high, it may extract nutrients from bones and other tissues to correct the balance. See *Alkaline Diet*

Acid-Base Balance – See *Acid/Alkaline Balance*

Acid Reflux – A disease caused when hydrochloric acid from the stomach backs up into the oesophagus, causing symptoms such as heartburn, bloating, and nausea. There is some evidence that acid reflux may be an *autoimmune disease*. In addition, research shows that eating a diet low in carbohydrates may help to eliminate acid reflux. See *Low Carb*

Acne – A skin disease very common in adolescents. While some older studies discounted the link between diet and acne, more recent research indicates that the *Western Pattern diet* is very likely at the root of acne. *Loren Cordain* has conducted studies that support this theory, as have other researchers around the world, based on *gut flora* imbalances, *inflammation*, a diet of foods with a high *glycaemic index.*, consuming dairy, and wheat. Eating a *Paleo diet* can help to reduce or eliminate acne.

Activated Almonds – *Almonds* that have been long-soaked in salt water, then long-dried at low temperatures (below 70C), breaking down the enzyme inhibitors and phytates, thereby improving digestion and increasing nutritional value. See *Soaking*, *Phytates*

Activity – See *Physical Activity*

Adipose Tissue – A clinical term used to describe body fat. See *Fat Loss*

Adrenal Fatigue – A syndrome typified by *chronic fatigue* and caused by under-functioning *adrenal glands.* Some symptoms of adrenal fatigue include memory loss, inability to concentrate, muscle pain, headaches, and joint pain. Our hunter-gatherer ancestors typically dealt with acute stress from the occasional flight-or-fight situation. In the modern era, non-stop chronic stress can lead to the adrenal glands always firing, resulting in burnout.

Adrenal Glands, *adrenals* – Located on top of the kidneys, these glands help the body maintain energy levels and manage *stress.*

Aflatoxins – Moulds (U.S. molds), a type of *mycotoxin,* which include certain species of fungi that are highly toxic and potent carcinogens. They thrive in warm, moist environments and may grow on stored *nuts* and *grains,* peanuts, *olive oil,* and in the milk of animals that eat contaminated food.

See *Toxins, Carcinogenic, Legumes*

Agave – A sweetener derived from agave juice and used as a sugar substitute. Agave has a lower *glycaemic index* than refined *sugar* does, so is arguably a better choice. However, if you are trying to lose weight, suffer from *Metabolic Syndrome*, or are pre-diabetic or *diabetic*, then it should be avoided. Agave is used in many Paleo dessert recipes.

Agricultural Revolution – Any period characterised by significant changes or developments in the field of agriculture. The agricultural revolution which happened around 10,000 BC marked the beginning of the human cultivation of crops. Instead of consuming foods we would typically hunt, gather or scavenge, we began to cultivate the soil, grow crops (including previously inedible or difficult to digest grains) and domesticate animals for livestock. The invention of the modern plough and other farming equipment sparked further agricultural revolutions in the eighteenth and nineteenth centuries. Some people, including Professor Jared Diamond of the University of California, Los Angeles, believe that agriculture as a whole has been detrimental to the human race. Diamond argues in his book *Guns, Germs,* *and Steel: The Fate of Human Societies* that since the Agricultural Revolution, human beings have been sick and malnourished. See *Neolithic*

AIP – See *Autoimmune Protocol*

Air Squat – A squat performed using just bodyweight as opposed to using additional weight. Air Squat example - *http://bit.ly/FE-Squat*

ALA (Alpha-Linolenic Acid) – See *Essential Fatty Acids*

Alcohol – Although there is some evidence to suggest slight health benefits when consumed in moderation, alcohol is calorie-dense but nutritionally void. There is overwhelming evidence that alcohol is the cause of more than sixty different medical conditions, with 4 per cent of all diseases attributable to alcohol globally. Here are a few little-known facts. Alcohol:

- Promotes the excretion of calcium from the bones
- Reduces *vitamin D* and *magnesium* function
- Reduces the ability to burn fat by up to 70 per cent
- Affects *blood sugar* metabolism

- Increases secretion of *cortisol,* while decreasing *testosterone* production
  Causes increased cortisol and decreased testosterone to last up to twenty-four hours after drinking
- Suppresses nighttime *human growth hormone* (hGH) by 70 per cent, accelerating the ageing process

Alkaline Diet – A diet based on the theory that we should consume mainly alkaline foods rather than acidic foods to ensure we maintain an *acid/alkaline balance*, or balanced blood pH, which leads to better health. In general, animal products and grains are acid-forming while *fruits* and *vegetables* are alkali-forming. The fundamental flaws behind this diet is that:

1. It is the kidneys' role to regulate blood pH
2. There are no observational or interventional *clinical trials* supporting the theory

However, there is likely to be an overall improvement in one's diet due to an increase in fruit and vegetable consumption when compared to the SAD (*Standard American Diet*).

Alkaloids – A chemical compound of plant origin composed of nitrogen, carbon, hydrogen and oxygen.

Most alkaloids are usually bitter and are present in the plant to prevent animals from eating it. Alkaloids have a pronounced effect on the nervous system of humans and other mammals, and many are used as drugs. Examples include _nicotine_, _caffeine_, morphine and cocaine. Alkaloids can be fatally toxic to humans too for example, atropine and strychnine.

Allergies – An immune reaction to any substance to which the body has enhanced sensitivity. Examples include plant pollen, dust, and particular foods. The _Paleo diet_ may help with food allergies because many of the most common food allergens (_peanuts_, _dairy_, _wheat_, and _soya_) are not part of the _Paleo diet_, it can also decrease chronic _systemic inflammation_ which may lower sensitivity to allergens.

Almonds – _Nuts_ that are high in _potassium_ and _magnesium_, _minerals_ important in regulating nerve function and known to lower blood pressure. Almonds are also high in _biotin_, which is necessary to build healthy fats in the skin. These fats keep the skin supple and moist and can prevent the skin from becoming flaky and irritated. Diets low in biotin can impair the production of *insulin*. Researchers from Pennsylvania State University (U.S.) report that a handful of almonds a day can lower LDL cholesterol whilst increasing HDL cholesterol levels in adults with elevated LDL levels. See *Cholesterol*

American Dietetic Association (ADA) – The largest organisation of food and nutrition professionals in the United States. They are now known as the Academy of Nutrition and Dietetics (AND) and are currently sponsored by Coca-Cola and PepsiCo.

Amino Acids – The building blocks of *protein*.

AMRAP – A common *Crossfit* term meaning 'as many rounds or reps as possible'. It refers to a workout that requires completing as many exercises as possible within a given timeframe.

Ancestral Health Symposium (AHS) – An annual three-day event in the United States that began in 2011 and is organised by the Ancestral Health Society. Their purpose is to bring together healthcare providers and scientists to discuss current health issues from an evolutionary standpoint. A sister event takes place in New Zealand in October 2015.

Antibacterials – See *Antibiotics*

Antibiotics (*antibacterials*) – A category of medicines used to treat or prevent bacterial infections. They do not work against infections, such as the common cold, that are caused by viruses. Nearly 50 per cent of all antibiotics are used on *factory farms* to compensate for crowded conditions and are prescribed routinely whether the animals require them or not. Excessive antibiotic use can lead to gut *dysbiosis*.

Antibiotic Resistance – A state where bacteria become resistant to certain *antibiotics*. Antibiotic resistance occurs over time when bacteria survive the antibiotic and reproduce strains that are not affected by it, which in turn leads to certain diseases becoming more difficult to treat. One cause of antibiotic resistance has been due to the unnecessary use of antibiotics. The director-general of the *World Health Organisation*, Dr Margaret Chan, warned in 2011 of an era in the not-too-distant future *"in which* *many common infections will no longer have a cure and, once again, kill unabated.*"

Antibodies – See *Immunoglobulin*

Antigen – Any substance, whether created by or introduced from outside the body, that the body detects as harmful, thereby triggering an *immune response*.

Anti-inflammatory – The ability of a substance to reduce *inflammation*.

Anti-inflammatory Foods – The key concepts are that constant inflammation in the body leads to ill health and that eating to avoid constant inflammation promotes better health, helping to ward off disease. Some examples of anti-inflammatory foods include *ginger, turmeric, green tea, oily fish*, pomegranate, and *garlic*. Foods that promote inflammation include *grains, dairy*, sugar, *alcohol, trans fats* and excess *omega-6 fatty acids*.

Antinutrient – A compound, natural or synthetic, that inhibits the absorption of nutrients by the body. Grains, legumes and other plant foods contain chemicals designed to protect them from being eaten or to remain intact while obtaining nutrients from the host as they pass through the digestive tract. Some of these proteins are broken down by cooking, sprouting and fermenting, but others are resistant to these procedures, which leads to gut irritation and inflammation. The most common examples are *lectins, phytates, protease inhibitors, oxalates, goitrogens, saponins,* and *tannins.* The *Paleo diet* helps the body to absorb more of the vital nutrients it needs to function well because the diet reduces or eliminates antinutrient foods. Eating a wide variety of plant foods is also a failsafe to ensure that you will not overload on a particular antinutrient. See *Nutrient Interaction*

Antioxidants – Molecules that inhibit oxidation reactions from other molecules known as '*free radicals*' which are a type of molecule that can lead to cell damage or even cell death. Some common antioxidants include *vitamin A, vitamin C, vitamin E,* and *polyphenols.* Antioxidants may help to prevent diseases such as cancer, heart disease, and *autoimmune diseases.* Many *fruits* and *vegetables* contain high levels of antioxidants, which are hugely responsible for health benefits based on their consumption. They are also better sources of antioxidants than are *supplements*. Studies are inconclusive when it comes to providing substantial evidence on antioxidant supplements impacting disease. See *Phytonutrients*

Arrhythmia – An abnormal rhythm of the heart that can cause the heart to pump less efficiently and could potentially be fatal. See *Caffeine*

Artificial Sweeteners – Any synthetic sugar substitute, including aspartame, sucralose, saccharin, and acesulfame K. Artificial sweeteners are zero-calorie or low-calorie substitutes used by the food industry. Some sweeteners, such as sucralose, are an incredible 600 times sweeter than *sugar* and can stimulate the area of the brain that creates a desire for more. Significant amounts of research indicate that many of them are *carcinogenic, neurotoxic* and can cause harmful side effects, including *hypertension* and birth defects. See *Sweeteners*

Aspartame – See *Artificial Sweeteners*

Atkins Diet – A popular *low-carb*, high-protein, high-fat diet popularised by Dr Charles Atkins. The book *Dr.*

Atkins' Diet Revolution was a 1972 *New York Times* bestseller.

Autoimmune Disease (Autoimmune Disorders) – A disease in which the body's *immune system* attacks and destroys healthy body tissue by mistake. Some of the more common ones include *type I diabetes, Crohn's disease, Hashimoto's thyroiditis, rheumatoid arthritis, coeliac disease, Graves' disease, multiple sclerosis*, and *lupus*. The severity of symptoms can vary, as well as the durations of attacks which can last days, weeks, or months. Attacks can be followed by periods of reduced or no symptoms known as *remissions*. A return of the disease is termed a *relapse*, however, the disease may continue to get worse without periods of remission. There are no cures for autoimmune diseases however the *Paleo diet* can help to reduce the impact of the disease and to decrease systems, especially during flare-ups by eliminating many of the foods such as *grains, dairy*, and *processed foods* that cause the immune system to turn on itself. See *Autoimmune Protocol*

Autoimmune Disorders – See *Autoimmune Diseases*

Autoimmune Protocol (AIP) – A specialised version of the *Paleo diet* that helps people with *autoimmune disorders* to manage their disease and its symptoms. The AIP works by eliminating foods that can cause *inflammation* in the gut, such as *alcohol*, **eggs**, *grains*, *dairy*, *legumes*, *seeds*, *nuts* and foods that are in the *nightshade* family — this is one identifiable cause of autoimmune disease — and promoting foods that are anti-inflammatory, such as *bone broth* and *oily fish*. Currently more than eighty different *autoimmune diseases* have been identified.

See *Leaky Gut Syndrome*

B

"TAKE CARE OF YOUR BODY. IT'S THE ONLY
PLACE YOU HAVE TO LIVE."

—JIM ROHN

B12 – See *Vitamin B12*

Bacon – A pork product made from either the side or the belly of a pig. It is often smoked or cured. Avoid commercial bacon with added *nitrates*, *nitrites* and other ingredients of concern, which comes from factory-raised (*CAFO*) animals. Instead, choose bacon from naturally reared and *pastured* pigs.

Balance – A physical ability that uses significant brain power, as it involves vast amounts of information from different sources, including the eyes, muscles, and balance mechanisms in the inner ear. The ability to balance deteriorates starting in our thirties because the communication between the muscles and the *motor cortex* deteriorates. In simple terms, *use it or lose it*. See *Proprioception*

Barefoot Running – A natural response to the conventional running shoe industry's idea that we need heavily cushioned running shoes and from researchers investigating whether running shoes increase the likelihood of injury rather than prevent them. The hypothesis is that wearing running shoes detrimentally changes the way we run by increasing the probability of heel striking and by applying forces to the body that increase the chances of injury. Using *minimalist shoes* or going barefoot means you get closer to your natural stride with a midfoot or forefoot strike. Also, the stresses are applied to the parts of the body that have evolved to deal with them.

There is limited scientific evidence to support this hypothesis, but there are many anecdotal stories of reduced injuries to the knees, shins, and ankles and of people doing well with barefoot or minimalist running. The transition to barefoot running should take place over several weeks or months to reduce the likelihood of discomfort or injury.

Barefoot Shoes –
See *Minimalist Shoes*, *Barefoot Running*

Basil – A *herb* rich in *vitamin A*, *vitamin C*, *vitamin K*, *magnesium*, *iron*, *potassium*, and *calcium*. Contains anti-inflammatory and anti-ageing properties.

Basal Metabolic Rate (BMR) – Your BMR is a measurement of your body's use of energy and is usually interpreted as the minimum level of calories your body needs per day at rest to maintain normal bodily functions. It changes with age, height, weight, gender, muscle mass, levels of body fat, and levels of activity. See *Metabolism*

Beans – See *Legumes*

Benefits of the Paleo Diet – Based on *clinical trials*, personal observation, and a vast array of anecdotal evidence, the *Paleo lifestyle* has a positive impact on many of the *lifestyle diseases* plaguing Western society.

It can improve:

- bone density through increased levels of *micronutrient* intake
- *insulin sensitivity*, as more foods are eaten with lower *glycaemic loads*
- *bioavailability* of the required *minerals*
- digestion through improved *gut flora*
- nutrient absorption (vitamins A, D, E and K are *fat-soluble vitamins*; low-fat diets reduce the absorption of these vitamins)

- sleep quality by eliminating or reducing beverages containing *caffeine* and *alcohol,* which affect the quantity and quality of deep and *REM sleep*

It can reduce:

- *hypertension* by reducing sodium (*salt*) intake, resulting in a better sodium/potassium ratio
- body fat, thereby improving body composition
- *inflammation* by raising the body's *anti-inflammatory* profile through an improved *omega-3:6 ratio*
- exposure to food *toxins* and pollutants through the choosing of organic and naturally reared products

Additionally, the Paleo diet can allow remission and management of certain diseases (such as *coeliac disease,* type I and type II diabetes, *rheumatoid arthritis, Crohn's disease, irritable bowel syndrome,* and ulcerative colitis) without drugs.

Beta Carotene – See *Vitamin A*

Beverages – Should be mainly *water.* Other options include unsweetened green and white *teas* and herbal teas like peppermint, chamomile (camomile), and other non-fruit teas. *Coconut water,* a natural isotonic beverage, is also a popular choice. See *Beverages to Avoid*

Big 8 – The most common food allergens: *wheat, dairy, soya, peanuts, nuts, fish, shellfish,* and *eggs* which according to the U.S. Food and Drug Administration cause over 90 per cent of all food allergies. Peanuts are the most common food allergen.

Big Agra – Describes both the world's largest agricultural companies and their philosophies about food production. Large agricultural companies control most of the planet's arable land. In some countries such as the United States, they genetically alter crops and seeds to produce higher yields. These plants, known as *'genetically modified organisms'* (*GMOs*), form a significant percentage of the ingredients in *processed foods*. Evidence has linked them to diseases such as *cancer, depression, fatigue,* and infections.

Big Pharma – Refers to the largest companies in the pharmaceutical industry. Most of these enterprises have annual revenues of £1.5 billion or more and spend more than £300,000 per year on research and development. Big Pharma wields significant influence over the prescription drug market worldwide. Through Internet, radio, print and television advertising, they promote the use of drugs to treat diseases and have contributed to a persistent belief that medications are the solution to every health problem. The U.S. and New Zealand are the only two countries in the world where the governments allow prescription drugs to be advertised on TV.

Bioavailability – Refers to the availability of a nutrient to be absorbed during digestion. For example, *omega-3* supplements have a lower degree of bioavailability than does a piece of fish, such as wild-caught salmon, that is high in omega-3. Factors that may affect bioavailability include supplement formulations, gut health, disease, and other foods consumed at the same time. See *Supplements*

Biodynamics (Biodynamic Farming) – An approach to agriculture that strives to imbue it with an awareness of the ecological, ethical, and spiritual repercussions of how we produce food. This includes treating crops with compost and manure as opposed to chemical fertilisers and looking at plants, soil, and animals as part of a unified system. See *Organic, Sustainability*

Bioelectrical Impedance Analysis (BIA) – A method that measures body composition by sending a low, safe, electrical current through the body via a set of scales. The current passes freely through fluids, organs, and muscle tissue but encounters resistance (impedance) when it passes through fat tissue. The resistance to the current by the fat tissue is termed *'bioelectrical impedance'*. This takes into account your height, gender, and weight, and the scales then compute your ***body fat percentage***. This method is more reliable than a ***BMI*** measurement. Try to take the test the same time of day on each occasion to improve accuracy. It is not 100 per cent accurate, but it gives you a baseline from which to monitor your progress.

Biohacking – The practice of merging the study of biology with the so-called hacker mentality. The ultimate goal is to improve human health and longevity through the use of technology, nutrition, and medical devices. Examples of biohacking are strategies for ***sleep*** and diet optimisation.

See ***Wearable Tech***

Biophilia – A term popularised by Edward O. Wilson in his book of the same name. The word *biophilia* means 'love of life', but Wilson defined it as a human desire to have an innate affinity with other life forms. Being outdoors and observing nature is a great stress release. Research published in *Environment and Behaviour* found that viewing natural scenes can reduce your *stress* levels.

Biotin – See *Vitamin B7*

Bisphenol A – See *BPA*

Black Pepper – A *spice* that is a source of manganese, *vitamin K*, copper, *iron*, chromium, and *calcium*. It also acts as a *thermogenic*, which means it increases metabolic rate. Piperine, a constituent in black pepper, fights the development of new fat cells, which may help in fat loss efforts – it also increases the absorption of nutrients.

Blood Glucose – See *Blood Sugar*

Blood Pressure – A measure of the pressure of the blood against the walls of the arteries. This value is presented as two numbers in fraction form, such as 124/82, for example. The top number (systolic) represents the pressure when the heart contracts to pump blood to the body. The bottom number (diastolic) represents the pressure when the heart relaxes between beats. Blood pressure of around 110/70 mmHg (millimetres of mercury) is considered optimal for adults. A normal systolic reading would range from 90 to 120 mmHg and a normal diastolic reading from 60 to 80 mmHg. See *Hypertension, Hypotension*

Blood Sugar (blood glucose) – A measure of how much glucose is in a person's blood. The term for blood sugar that is too high is hyperglycaemia; blood sugar that is too low is called hypoglycaemia. Persistent hyperglycaemia may develop into *type II diabetes*. The *Paleo diet* may help to maintain healthy blood sugar levels by reducing the consumption of foods with a high *glycaemic load*.

Blood Tests – See *Blood Work*

Blood Type Diet – A diet based on the premise that a person's blood type dictates how we react to foods and *toxins*. The Blood Type Diet works on the theory that the *lectins* in various foods are reactive with particular blood types. The key flaw behind this diet is that there are no *clinical trials* supporting the theory.

Blood Work – The name for a group of *blood tests* that are taken together. Some common blood tests determine *cholesterol* and *blood sugar* levels while others test for mineral levels or evidence of disease. Many people who commence the *Paleo diet* get blood work done to track their results over a period to determine whether their dietary and lifestyle changes are beneficial. Most blood work may need to be performed in a fasted state for accurate results. Aim for a twelve-hour fast.

Some common tests include:

- FBC: Full blood count – A full blood count gives valuable information about the kinds and numbers of cells in the blood, especially red blood cells and white blood cells

- CBC: Complete blood count (or BC: blood count) – A complete blood count is the term used in the U.S. for full blood count.

- Blood/Serum glucose: A screening for the level of glucose in the blood.

  o Conventional range:
    - Standard International Units: 3.61–6.38 mmol/L
    - Standard U.S. units: 65–115 mg/dL
  o Optimal range:
    - Standard International Units: 3.9–4.99 mmol/L
    - Standard U.S. units: 70–90 mg/dL

- Haemoglobin A1C (***HbA1c***)
  o Conventional range:
    - Standard International Units: < 0.07
    - Standard U.S. units: less than 7%
  o Optimal range:
    - Standard International Units: 0.041–0.057
    - Standard U.S. units: 4.1–5.7%

- Total Cholesterol: A blood measurement of all the cholesterol found in the body – LDL cholesterol, HDL cholesterol, VLDL and triglycerides.
  o Conventional range:
    - Standard International Units: 3.36–5.2 mmol/L
    - Standard U.S. units: 130–200 mg/dL
  o Optimal range:

- Standard International Units: 3.9–5.7 mmol/L
- Standard U.S. units: 150–220 mg/dL

- ***C-Reactive Protein***
  - Conventional range:
    - < 5.0
  - Optimal range:
    - < 1.0 (detected using a high-sensitivity C-reactive protein [hs-CRP] test)

- Sodium (serum):
  - Standard International Units: 135-145 mmol/L
  - Standard U.S. units: 135-145 mEq/L

- Vitamin D3: Ensure you get tested for the ***vitamin D*** marker *25-hydroxy vitamin D* also referred to as '*25(OH)D*' which is the most accurate way to measure how much vitamin D is in your body and work with a practitioner to determine the right dosage.

- HDL cholesterol (high-density lipoprotein): Lipoproteins that carry cholesterol from the arteries to the liver.

- LDL cholesterol (low-density lipoprotein): Lipoproteins made by the liver that carry cholesterol and ***fat-soluble vitamins*** from the liver to the cells. It is usually calculated from the following formula:

LDL cholesterol = total cholesterol − (HDL + triglycerides/5)

- VLDL: Very-low-density lipoproteins made by the liver. A VLDL particle is an LDL particle that contains the highest amount of triglycerides.

Cholesterol ratios usually provide more useful information than absolute values in isolation. Some important ratios are:

- Total cholesterol/HDL ratio: Optimal range is below 4.0

- HDL/LDL ratio: Optimal range is above 0.4

- Triglyceride/HDL ratio: Optimal range is below one as long as HDL is high and triglycerides are low

Blue Blockers – See *Sleep Tips*

BMI (Body Mass Index) – A calculation used to determine the percentage of body fat in a human body. The formula is a person's weight divided by the height squared. For example, if your height is 1.92 metres and your weight is 90 kilograms, the calculation would be 90/(1.92*1.92) = 24.41. A BMI of 25 or above is classified as *overweight*, and a BMI of 30 or above indicates *obesity*. The BMI statistics do not differentiate between muscle mass, fat mass, and body shape. So, for example, a healthy athlete with a muscular build could be classified as overweight or even obese based on the formula above. It is worth stating that, even though, this is not the best method for measuring total body fat, it is a very quick and non-intrusive guide. For more accuracy, other methods such as *bioelectrical impedance analysis* and *body fat calipers* should be considered.

Body Composition – Refers to the ratio between lean body mass and fat mass. See *Body Fat Percentage*

Body Fat Calipers – A tool used to measure skin folds at various points on the body to calculate how much subcutaneous fat (fat under the skin) a person has. These numbers are entered into a formula to calculate the *body fat percentage*. Normally a personal trainer or health professional is required to perform this task, but there are self-measurement body fat calipers available so you can test yourself reliably.

Body Fat Percentage (total body fat) – A reading that estimates the percentage of the body that is fat. Body fat levels that are too low are just as damaging as fat levels that are too high. Here is a breakdown of different levels of body fat percentage:

Women (by per cent)

- Essential fat: 10–13
- Athletic: 14–20
- Average: 21–24
- Above average: 25–30
- Overweight: 31–34
- Obese: 35–39
- Morbidly obese: > 40

Men (by per cent)

- Essential fat: 2–5
- Athletic: 6–13
- Average: 14–17
- Above average: 18–25
- Overweight: 26–30
- Obese: 31–35
- Morbidly obese: > 36

Three popular methods to determine body fat percentage are **BMI**, **bioelectrical impedance analysis**, and **body fat calipers.** See **Skinny Fat, Obesity, Overweight**

Bodyweight Exercises – Exercise that is performed using solely the weight of the body as resistance. For example, during a press-up (push-up) or a pull-up, your own bodyweight is supported throughout the movement. See *Strength*

Boiling – Most people assume boiling foods such as *vegetables* to be detrimental to maintaining the food's nutrients, as it reduces vitamin levels. It is true that half the *water soluble vitamins* in, say, carrots will be destroyed, but other nutrients become more plentiful with boiling. For example, *vegetables* that have boiled for ten minutes have the highest levels of carotenoids (*antioxidants*) when compared to raw or steamed vegetables. See *Cooking*

Bone Broth – A broth made from the bones of animals. When properly prepared, bone broth is rich in *minerals*, including *calcium* and *magnesium*, and it also contains collagen and glucosamine, which promote joint health. Also known as *meat tea* or *beef tea* in the UK.

To make bone broth, put 1kg (2 lbs) of bones into a stewing pot with vegetables of your choice (for example, celery, carrots, onion). Add *herbs and spices* (for example, *thyme, garlic, rosemary,* and *black pepper*). Cover with water and simmer on low heat. Cook a minimum of four hours for chicken or fish bones, six hours for beef bones.

Bone Density – A measure of bone mineral content (*calcium* and other *minerals*), used to determine bone health and to diagnose *osteoporosis*. Research has shown that exercise and the development of muscle tissue are related to stronger, healthier bones. Bone mass declines after age 35, making you more vulnerable to fractures as you get older. The accelerated decline of bone mass accelerates after the menopause. Help to reduce this risk by doing enough weight-bearing activities and *exercise*, increasing levels of *micronutrient* intake through food, avoiding smoking, excessive drinking, and getting sufficient levels of *vitamin D*.

Bone Marrow – A fatty and nutrient-dense substance found in the centre of bones. Bone marrow contains stem cells, which boost immunity and help with blood clotting. It is also high in collagen, which aids digestion and can heal the body, including healing damage in the gastrointestinal tract. It is important to consume bone marrow from animals that are *pastured* and not those that are *grain-fed* or *factory-raised.*

Bone Mass – See *Bone Density*

Bone Stock – See *Bone Broth*

BPA (Bisphenol A) – In 2010 Canada became the first country to ban BPA for food product containers. In 2012, consumer pressure led to the European Union banning plastic baby feeding bottles that contain BPA, and there are discussions to ban BPA in all plastics that come into contact with food. Several U.S. states have banned BPA for baby-feeding containers.

The *Food and Drug Administration* (FDA) announced in April 2012 that it would not ban BPA in canned foods. Exposure can be reduced by avoiding plastic bottles containing BPA and instead using glass or stainless steel bottles. Use microwave-safe plates and glass to microwave foods and beverages. Reduce the purchase of packaged, processed, and canned foods and drinks, and avoid using plastic for food storage unless it is labelled as BPA-free. BPA has been linked to prostate, breast, and other cancers as well as brain and nerve damage in young children. See *Plastics*

BPA-Free – Designates a product free of *plastic* made with *BPA.*

Brazil Nuts – *Nuts* that are high in *selenium, calcium,* and *magnesium.* The *minerals* in Brazil nuts support muscle function, immune function, and bone health.

Breakfast – Many Paleo breakfasts include *eggs* or other animal protein as well as *fruits, nuts,* and *vegetables.* Especially convenient are leftovers from the night before. Here is a sample breakfast made with coconut milk, use organic and fresh ingredients where possible.

Coconut Surprise Muesli (serves two)

Mix:

- Coconut milk (350ml/12 fl oz.)
- Two bananas (sliced)
- Two handfuls of *walnuts*
- One handful of *cashews*
- Shredded *coconut*

Breathing – Most people take shallow breaths using just the chest, but when you take the time to inhale and exhale deeply, known as *diaphragmatic breathing*, you get more oxygen in and more **toxins** out. This type of breathing reduces **blood pressure**, encourages relaxation, and can be used to manage **stress** by strengthening the **parasympathetic nervous system**. Here is a simple breathing exercise that can be used to develop this technique.

1. Start by clearing your mind and focussing only on your breathing. Feel the air come into your lungs and go out of your lungs.
2. Close your mouth and take a deep breath in through the nose for four seconds.
3. Hold that breath for eight seconds.
4. Breathe out through the mouth, slowly and controlled, for eight seconds.
5. Repeat steps 1 through 4 four times.
6. Finish by breathing normally, but continue to focus on breathing technique.

Brown Fat – Deposits of brown **adipose tissues** found in the body. This kind of fat burns calories by turning energy into heat when we are exposed to the cold. Japanese researchers at Hokkaido University found that spending two hours a day at a temperature of 17°C (63°F) for six weeks lowered body fat by an average of 5.2 per cent and increased activity of brown fat by 58 per cent.

Bulletproof Coffee – A mixture of special coffee that is free of *mycotoxins* and with butter and *MCT* oils added. Proponents of bulletproof coffee say that the fat helps keep full those who skip breakfast, helps with *weight loss* and provides an energy boost. Detractors counter that it is unhealthy to replace a nutritious breakfast with something that has such little nutritional content.
See *Caffeine*

Butter – See *Dairy*

C

"**T**HE HUMAN BODY IS THE BEST PICTURE OF THE HUMAN SOUL."

—LUDWIG WITTGENSTEIN

Cachexia – The medical term for extreme *weight loss* when not trying to lose weight. Other symptoms include fatigue, loss of appetite, loss of muscle, and bone mass. Cachexia is often present in patients with HIV/AIDS, *cancer, multiple sclerosis, autoimmune disorders*, and other diseases. See *Sarcopenia*

Cadmium – One of only three *heavy metal* contaminants, along with *lead* and *mercury*, for which the European Commission has set maximum permitted contamination levels in food.

Caffeine – An *alkaloid* psychoactive drug found in coffee, *chocolate*, and other foods. Coffee contains *antioxidants*, which neutralise free radicals. Caffeine also boosts brain function, elevates *metabolism*, and increases athletic performance. It blocks the adenosine receptors that cause tiredness. However, it can also irritate the stomach, increase the *resting heart rate* by 10 to 15 beats per minute, increase the force per heartbeat, and lead to *arrhythmias*. Caffeine can also disrupt the quality of *sleep* by reducing rapid eye movement (*REM*) and deep sleep, the time when your body recuperates. Some people are more susceptible to these side effects than others. Caffeine has a half-life of six to eight hours, so even 100 milligrams of caffeine from a cup of coffee first thing in the morning can affect deep sleep that night, as 25 milligrams will still be in your system at bedtime.

Caffeine Content – Levels of caffeine in various foods and beverages:

- Cup of white tea – 6 mg
- Cup of green tea – 15 mg
- Cup of black tea – 50 mg
- Can of Coca-Cola – 32 mg
- Can of Diet Coke – 45 mg
- Can of Red Bull – 80 mg
- Can of Relentless – 160 mg
- Can of No Fear – 200 mg
- Large latte – 160 mg
- Single espresso shot – 75 mg
- Short coffee – 180 mg
- Tall coffee – 260 mg
- Grande coffee – 330 mg
- Vente coffee – 415 mg
- 100 g (3.5 oz.) of dark chocolate – 100 mg

Caffeine Withdrawal – When regular drinkers of caffeinated drinks stop drinking caffeine, they may suffer from headaches and fatigue and feel irritable for several days while their body adjusts.

CAFO (Concentrated Animal Feeding Operation) – A production process that concentrates large quantities of animals into confined spaces, also known as *factory raised*. See *Factory Farmed*, *Organic*

Calcium – An important *mineral* for the human body. There is more calcium in the body than any other *mineral*, and the body requires *magnesium*, phosphorous, *vitamin D*, and *vitamin K* to absorb it. Calcium has several important functions including maintaining healthy bones and teeth. When we remove *dairy* products from our diet, we rely on obtaining calcium from eating foods that are calcium-rich, such as *dark greens* like kale and spring/fresh greens (collard greens) as well as *nuts*. Fish with edible bones, such as sardines and pilchards, and seafood such as oysters are great sources, too. *Salt* is thought to accelerate the loss of calcium from the bones, and *alcohol* and *caffeinated* *drinks* can reduce the amount of calcium absorbed, too. See *Bone Density*

Calorie – A unit of heat, measuring how much energy it takes to warm one kilogram of water by one degree Celsius. Food manufacturers and nutritionists use the calorie to express the specific amount of food energy contained in a meal or a serving of a particular food. Many diets use calorie counting as a tool to manage food intake. The *Paleo diet* does not rely on calorie counting. Instead, weight management and *weight loss* usually occur because the foods allowed on the *Paleo diet* are lower in high *glycaemic* carbohydrates and increase satiety (*feeling full*) because of increased protein and fat content. See *Calories In vs Calories Out*

Calories In vs Calories Out (Energy Balance) – *Conventional wisdom* tells us that if you restrict calories and/or increase activity levels that exceed your daily energy requirements, you can (and usually will) lose weight. But there are some who don't eat too much (or indeed eat too little), and yet they still have issues with managing a healthy body composition. There are also those who exercise excessively, and they, too, can have issues with maintaining a healthy *body fat percentage*. In 2004, biochemist Eugene Fine proposed that the concept of '*a calorie is a calorie*' violates the second law of thermodynamics and that the body does not metabolise *macronutrients* in the same way. Factors contributing to weight gain include (but are not limited to) the type of foods consumed, hormonal imbalances, *insulin sensitivity*, levels of *stress*, and *sleep* deprivation.

Cancer – There is evidence to suggest that our hunter-gatherer ancestors did not suffer from cancer, or at least had much lower rates. Leading a healthy lifestyle can help lower the risk of developing certain cancers. Research shows that the risk of cancer can be reduced by ingesting less refined carbohydrates and fewer *processed foods*, not smoking, having sufficient *vitamin D* levels, drinking less alcohol, reducing exposure to *carcinogenic* environmental toxins such as asbestos, being physically active (which can reduce the risk especially of cancers of the colon, breast, prostate, pancreas, and lung) and maintaining a healthy weight.

Candida – A *yeast* that lives on the skin and in mucous membranes. Some candida in the body is normal, but an overgrowth is the cause of many common fungal infections, including vaginal yeast infections and thrush. Candida is also a culprit in gut infections. The *Paleo diet* helps correct *gut imbalance* and may, therefore, help to eliminate *candidiasis*.

Candidiasis – a variety of infections caused by *candida* overgrowth, occurring most often in the mouth, respiratory tract or vagina.

Canola Oil – A cooking oil derived from the seeds of the rape plant. Because of its high levels of *omega-6* and *polyunsaturated fats* as well as the presence of erucic acid (a known *carcinogen*), canola oil is not recommended.

Carb Flu (also Low-Carb Flu) – Flu-like symptoms brought on by a switch from eating a diet high in carbohydrates to one low in carbohydrates. The body's adjustment to a new way of eating may cause fatigue and other symptoms. The *Paleo diet* is not a *low-carb* diet by design because it does not limit the amount of carbohydrates eaten, only the kinds of carbohydrates eaten. For those with metabolic problems, easing into the Paleo diet may be the answer to avoiding the Carb Flu.

Carbohydrates – Organic compounds found in sugars, starches, and dietary fibre. Carbohydrates are described as simple (e.g., glucose and saccharides) or complex (starches such as those in *sweet potatoes*). Refined carbohydrates relate to the high level of nutrient-depleting processing involved. Carbohydrates come mainly from plant-based foods. They are common sources of dietary fibre, *prebiotics*, and *essential nutrients* that are crucial for *gastrointestinal* health. The digestive process breaks down carbohydrates into glucose, which is the form of *sugar* transported and used by the body. This glucose is used immediately as energy, stored as glycogen in the liver, or stored as *adipose tissue*.

Modern convenience means we often substitute *fruits* and *vegetables* for *cereal grains*, *sugar*, and *dairy* as our primary forms of carbohydrate because of low cost, ease of preparation, and extended shelf life. *Fruits* and *vegetables* are often overlooked when individuals consider carbohydrate intake, but historically, our hunter-gatherer ancestors ate them as their primary source of carbohydrates. See *Low-Carb Diet, Protein, Fats*

Carcinogenic, carcinogens – A substance that either causes *cancer* or increases the chances that a person may develop cancer. Some common carcinogens are asbestos, *aflatoxins, alcohol,* and *tobacco.*

Casein – A *protein* found in *dairy* products. Casein proteins constitutes around 80 per cent of the proteins in milk and are responsible for most milk allergies. See *Whey, Casein Intolerance, Lactose Intolerance*

Casein Intolerance (See also *Food Intolerance*) – A dairy intolerance that occurs when an individual has problems breaking down casein. Symptoms of casein intolerance include:

- Bloating
- Vomiting
- Cramps
- Diarrhoea
- Constipation
- Skin problems

Cashews – Nuts that are a rich source of *magnesium*, phosphorus, copper, manganese, and *tryptophan*.

Causation – The relationship between cause and effect. The capacity of one variable to affect another. The first variable may lead the second to exist, or can influence the second variable to fluctuate. An observation may appear to establish a relationship (*correlation*) between the first and second variable. However, there may be a third variable that is responsible for the differences in the variables. Hence why causation is often confused with correlation when reviewing *research*.

Challenges – Any programme designed to challenge the body for a set period, usually thirty days. This can include dietary challenges such as Whole 30, a thirty-day regimen that eliminates *sugar*, *alcohol*, *grains*, *legumes*, *dairy*, and food additives to kick-start commencing the Paleo diet. See *Cognitive Dissonance*

Cheese – See *Dairy*

Chia Seeds – Seeds of the chia plant, a member of the mint family. Chia seeds are very high in ALA *omega-3* and fibre and are good sources of calcium, iron, and zinc. However, they also contain numerous **antinutrients**, such as **phytates**, that reduce their nutrient value.

Chives – A **herb** which is rich in vitamins **A, C** and contains vitamins **B6** and **K**. Aids **sleep**, muscle function, and cognitive function.

Chocolate (Dark) – Food that can be a healthy part of the **Paleo diet**. Make sure to choose a dark chocolate with a minimum of 70 per cent cocoa. In general, the darkest chocolate has the least amount of **sugar** and **dairy** added to it. A 100-gram serving of dark chocolate has more than half of the manganese, copper, **magnesium**, and **iron** your body needs on a daily basis. It is also highly **antioxidant** and helps promote circulatory health and brain function.

Cholesterol – A fatty molecule found in all cells of the body, used for a variety of purposes, including the manufacture of cell membranes, lining of the nerves, the production of steroid hormones such as **oestrogen** and **testosterone**, and to make Vitamin D when the skin is exposed to sunlight. There are two main types of cholesterol: low-density lipoproteins (LDL) known as 'bad' cholesterol, and high-density lipoproteins (HDL) or 'good' cholesterol. However, not all LDL is bad. It is the small, dense, atherogenic (promoting fatty deposits in the arteries) LDL that is problematic. This distinction is based on particle size and can be determined by advanced *blood work*. Very-low-density lipoproteins (VLDL) contain a high level of triglycerides. High quantities and large VLDL particles sizes are also associated with an increased risk of cardiovascular disease or stroke.

The human body manufactures all necessary cholesterol, but many foods contain cholesterol too, such as meat, poultry and eggs, however current research states that cholesterol from foods does not correlate with serum (blood) cholesterol levels in the body. *Conventional wisdom* says that high levels of total cholesterol contribute to heart disease, but the overwhelming evidence suggests that *inflammation* and other markers such as elevated *triglycerides* as a primary cause of coronary disease. The USDA has indicated it will accede to new research (February 2015) stating that there is no appreciable relationship between dietary cholesterol and cardiovascular disease. Its Dietary Guidelines Advisory Committee plans to no longer warn people to avoid eggs, meat and other cholesterol-loaded foods, claiming that *"Cholesterol is not a nutrient of concern for overconsumption."*

There is evidence that people with higher cholesterol levels live longer than people with lower cholesterol levels. In 2012, the *Journal of Evaluation in Clinical Practice* published a ten-year study of more than 52,000 women. The study found that women with high total levels of cholesterol i.e. above 6.98 mmol/L (270 mg/dL) were 30 per cent less likely to die from heart disease, a heart attack, or stroke than women with a normal total cholesterol level below 4.99 mmol/L (193 mg/dL) suggesting that high total cholesterol levels are not linked to poor heart health. In 2011, a study reviewing the association between low total cholesterol levels and cancer in the *Monthly Journal of the Association of Physicians* stated that studies of healthy people have shown low cholesterol as a risk marker for future cancer.

Because the **Paleo diet** reduces inflammation, reduces triglycerides, boosts the **immune system** and naturally raises your good cholesterol while reducing the small, dense LDL this mitigates the risk associated with cardiovascular disease. See *Fats*

Cholesterol Unit Conversion – In American literature, *cholesterol* is typically measured in milligrams per decilitre (mg/dL). To calculate a rough conversion to the standard international units of millimoles per litre (mmol/L), divide the American number by 40. For example, a total cholesterol of (U.S.) 200 mg/dL is roughly five mmol/L.

Chloride – See *Salt, Minerals*

Chromium – A micronutrient that may enhance *insulin* action and maintain normal *blood glucose* concentration and carbohydrate *metabolism*. A diet rich in *fruits* and *vegetables* should be sufficient to obtain adequate chromium. Broccoli, for example, is an excellent source of chromium. Chromium picolinate is the form generally taken as a supplement.

Chronic Cardio – A term that describes extended and intense cardio workouts at over 80 per cent of your maximum heart rate. In addition, working out at a high level of intensity for lengthy periods may harm the body because it keeps the body's *fight-or-flight* defence system in a constant state of readiness, contributing to chronic *stress*.

Chronic Disease – A long-term condition that can be controlled but not cured. According to the World Health Organisation, in the UK chronic diseases are projected to account for 85 per cent of all deaths. See *Lifestyle Disease*

Chronic Fatigue – A disorder that causes persistent exhaustion and does not go away with sleep or rest. Expected root causes include a viral infection, a compromised *immune system*, and hormonal imbalances.

Chronic Fatigue Syndrome (CFS) – See *Chronic Fatigue*

Chronic Inflammation – See *Inflammation*

Chronic Stress – See *Stress*

Circadian Rhythm – Any biological process that takes place over a twenty-four-hour period. Every cell in the body has its own daily circadian rhythm, or time when certain functions take place. There is a master circadian clock in the middle of the brain called the suprachiasmatic nucleus (SCN), which is regulated in part by the release of the hormone *melatonin* when darkness falls (helping us to feel sleepy) and by daylight, which suppresses melatonin in the morning. The SCN is comparable to the conductor of an orchestra and the peripheral clocks in the rest of the body are similar to orchestral musicians that are required to work in harmony.

Circadian rhythms dictate the body's production of *hormones* such as melatonin and *cortisol*, which help to regulate sleep patterns and manage *stress*. Outside stimuli, such as heat and light, may influence circadian rhythms. Disrupted circadian rhythms may be a contributing factor to diseases such as *diabetes*, *obesity*, and bipolar disorder and the reason we struggle with *jet lag* when travelling across several time zones.

Clinical Trials – A clinical trial is a *research* study that uses human volunteers to establish the answer to specific health questions, such as comparing one treatment with another or whether new medicines work as expected. The two types of clinical trials are interventional (these trials test whether therapies are safe and effective) or observational (these trials examine health issues in large groups of people).

Clean Fifteen – A list by the *EWG* of conventionally grown non-*organic fruits* and *vegetables* in the United States that are least likely to have pesticide residues. As of 2015 this list includes avocados, asparagus, cabbage, cantaloupe (British: honeydew melon), cauliflower, eggplant (British: aubergine), grapefruit, kiwis, mangoes, onions, papayas, pineapples, sweet corn, sweet peas, *sweet potatoes*. See *Dirty Dozen*

Cloves – A *spice* that can serve as a painkiller and antiseptic. Clove oil can be smeared on sore gums and toothache to numb the pain.

Coconut – Despite its name, the coconut is not a nut but rather an extremely versatile type of fruit known as a *drupe.* Coconut has become a Paleo staple due to its flexibility as a food source. Humans consume coconut in several different forms, including the flesh, coconut butter, coconut milk, coconut oil, coconut flour and coconut water.

Coconut Butter – A spread made from the flesh of the coconut similar to the way peanuts are used to make peanut butter.

Coconut Flour – Naturally *gluten-free*, contains no *phytates* that impede the absorption of *minerals*. Coconut flour is also higher in fibre and protein than other gluten-free flours such as almond flour.

Coconut Milk – A milky white liquid expressed from the grated flesh of brown coconut, can be used as a dairy substitute.

Coconut Oil – An oil that is rich in *antioxidants* and medium-chain fatty acids. Coconut oil has a high level of saturated fat (86 per cent) mainly in the form of lauric acid, a medium-chain saturated fatty acid, which helps to increase levels of HDL cholesterol. It is stable when heated, which makes it great for frying, and it is also a great moisturiser for the skin, scalp, and dry hair. Organic, cold-pressed **extra virgin or virgin** coconut oils are the least processed and the most nutritious. Refined coconut oil has less coconut smell and is usually less expensive than virgin or extra virgin coconut oil but can be less nutritious (containing fewer **phytonutrients**) due to the additional processing that occurs during manufacture, this can include bleaching, chemical solvents for oil extraction and high heat levels for deodorising.

Coconut Water – A refreshing, naturally isotonic clear drink obtained from inside a young, green coconut. Coconut water should be consumed in moderation because of a relatively high carbohydrate content. Drink fresh when possible, as cartoned or bottled coconut water may be made from concentrate, be **pasteurised** (which alters the taste and reduces nutrient content), and have artificial additives, sweeteners, and preservatives.

Coeliac Disease (U.S. Celiac) – An **autoimmune disease** in which the body's **immune system** forms **antibodies** to **gluten**. The immune system then attacks the intestinal lining. This can cause **weight loss**, malnutrition, **inflammation**, and a host of other symptoms including diarrhoea, constipation, nausea and vomiting, stomach cramps, bloating, fatigue, and frequent mouth ulcers. The onset of symptoms is weeks to years after gluten exposure. Coeliac disease is tested with a blood test that looks for the antibodies that your body produces in response to eating gluten. 76 per cent of people with the condition, remain undiagnosed. See **Cross-Reactivity, Non-Coeliac Gluten Sensitivity**

Coffee – See **Caffeine**

Cognitive Dissonance – A term used in psychology that refers to the discomfort you feel when you do something against your beliefs, the reaction is often guilt, disappointment, anger, or embarrassment. When this occurs people are motivated to reduce dissonance, this is usually achieved by justifying our actions (making excuses) or modifying our beliefs to match our actions. See **Confirmation Bias**

Cold Therapy – A therapy that uses various techniques to increase the skin's exposure to the cold for specific benefits. For example, taking a cold shower in the morning increases the levels of ***testosterone*** in the blood, which can aid in adding lean muscle mass, eradicating fat stores, and boosting energy. Cold showers may also strengthen the ***immune system*** and reduce ***DOMS*** after intense exercise.

Cold Thermogenesis – A way of using the body's generation of heat (thermogenesis) to increase ***metabolism*** and lose weight. The practice involves systematically exposing the body to cold temperatures in order to activate the body's fat-burning mechanisms.

Confirmation Bias – A tendency to research for or interpret information in a way that confirms one's preconceptions, ideas, and beliefs. It can lead to scientists such as Ancel Keys (see ***History of Fat***) to assign more weight to evidence that confirms a hypothesis and reject valid data which does not support it. See ***Cognitive Dissonance***

Conventional Wisdom – A term referring to any widely held idea or set of beliefs, whether it is true or not. Current conventional wisdom about nutrition is that the basis of the human diet should be high in *whole grains* and cereals and low in animal protein and saturated fat. However, the latest research tells us that the amount of saturated fat in the diet has no impact on heart health and that *trans fats*, refined carbohydrates, and sugar should be avoided.

Cooking – Heating food to render it more palatable, digestible, nutritious, and enjoyable. For example, cooking helps release both carbohydrates and proteins from food, and it also breaks down fibre, making it easier to absorb. It is difficult to know when humans started cooking their food, but archaeologists, palaeontologists, and food historians agree that widespread cooking first appeared between 100,000 and 125,000 years ago. The earliest cooking methods were probably roasting and boiling. In addition, cooking allowed *hunter-gatherers* to add foods to their diets that required cooking to make them edible. See *Boiling*

CoQ10 (Coenzyme Q10) – An enzyme that is present in every cell in the human body. Coenzymes work with the body's enzymes to help digest food, among other things.

CoQ10 is also an *antioxidant*, so it helps the body fight off infections. Most foods include some CoQ10, but *organ meats* contain the highest concentration.

Cordain, Loren – See *History of the Paleo Diet*, *Paleo Diet*, *Paleo Template*

Core – Refers to the muscles of the body's trunk, between the hips and the chest, which surround the spine and abdominals.

Coriander – A *herb*, also known as *cilantro*, or *dhania*. Rich in *vitamin A*, *vitamin C*, and *vitamin K* contains *potassium*, and traces of *iron* and *calcium*. Contains *anti-inflammatory* and antiseptic properties.

Corn-Fed – See *Grain-Fed*

Correlation – Used in *research* to denote an association or connection between two or more things. The correlated relationship is not necessarily connected with a root cause and effect (*causation*), yet many people make this incorrect assumption when interpreting statistical data.

For example, consider this true statement: *"In Scandinavia, more storks appear on the rooftops of families that have more children."* Does this mean families have more children because the storks delivered the babies? Alternatively, is it more plausible that the families with more children are likely to live in bigger houses with larger roofs and thus are more likely to have more storks on their rooftops? Or, is it that the more people there are within a household, the more opportunities there are for the storks to feed?

Cortisol – A hormone produced by the adrenal glands. Sometimes called *the **stress** hormone*, cortisol is the body's response to high-stress or fight-or-flight situations. It provides decreased pain sensitivity, increased energy, and other benefits to the body when needed. However, prolonged elevated cortisol, caused by long-term stress, lack of sleep, or excessive ***chronic cardio***, can lead to immune deficiencies, weight gain and is linked to conditions such as type II diabetes and hypertension. See *Laughter*

Cosmetics – See *Toiletries*

Crohn's Disease – An *autoimmune disease* affecting the bowels. Typically, the body's *immune system* recognizes healthy bacteria in the gut and does not attack it; with Crohn's disease, the body's immune system attacks healthy bacteria, causing chronic *inflammation* and ulceration.

Crossfit – A fitness programme that aims to improve all-round fitness based on ten components of fitness: cardiovascular/respiratory endurance, stamina, *strength*, flexibility, power, speed, agility, coordination, *balance*, and accuracy. Its adherents employ high-intensity training, Olympic lifting, rowing, running, and gymnastics.

Cross-Reactivity – A reaction between an *antigen* and an *antibody*. Cross-reactivity is what causes allergic reactions because the proteins in the allergen (for example, birch pollen) are too close to the proteins in a given food (apples.) *Coeliac disease* is an example of this: the body develops antigens against *gluten* and may then react to non-gluten substances as if they were gluten. A strict *Paleo diet*, especially *AIP*, is helpful in decreasing cross-reactivity because eliminating common food culprits may help to identify the foods that are causing the reaction. See *Yeast, Dairy*

CRP (C-Reactive Protein) – A vital part of the body's *immune system* as an inflammatory marker. CRP is part of an early response to infection or *inflammation*. High levels of CRP in the body indicate an infection or *immune disorder.* In *blood work*, CRP is used mainly as a marker for *systemic inflammation*; a high-sensitivity CRP (hs-CRP) test is usually used, as it can measure lower levels of CRP (less than 1 mg/dL). Adherence to a strict *Paleo diet* reduces inflammation and can alleviate immune dysfunction, thus lowering the body's CRP levels.

Cruciferous Vegetables – Vegetables that contain smelly sulphur compounds such as broccoli, Brussel sprouts, cauliflower, kale, onions, radishes, swede, turnips and watercress. These compounds are believed to help the *immune system* eliminate carcinogens. See *Leafy Green Vegetables*

D

"IF YOU WANT TO CONQUER THE ANXIETY OF LIFE, LIVE IN THE MOMENT, LIVE IN THE BREATH."

—AMIT RAY

Dairy – Milk and products made from milk. Dairy products include cream, milk, **yoghurt**, and cheese, among others. These products were not part of the human diet until the Agricultural or **Neolithic Revolution**. Dairy is a modern cultural adaptation and is not required after weaning; hence, most adults no longer produce enough of the enzyme **lactase** to break down the **lactose** in the milk, meaning they can be **lactose intolerant** to some degree. As such, dairy is arguably not an optimal food source for humans.

It is estimated that up to 75 per cent of adults worldwide have lost the ability to process lactose. This ranges from five per cent in northern Europe to 70 per cent in southern Europe to 90 per cent or more in some African and Asian countries. The issues are not just related to the carbohydrates in the milk (lactose), but also to the milk proteins (such as **casein** and **whey**) and hormones found in cow's milk. Research shows one of these hormones, called bovine insulin, is a possible cause of **type I diabetes** in children. Betacellulin, a protein growth factor, has potential links to **cancer** and **type II diabetes** and can be a contributing factor in *Leaky Gut Syndrome* as well as other *autoimmune diseases*. Dairy could also be a *cross-reacting* food to those who are sensitive to gluten.

Dance – A universal, widespread form of movement probably practiced by early humans as far back as 1.5 million years ago. Dance is a great way to develop coordination, agility, *balance*, muscular control, and *flexibility*.

Dehydration – The state of not having enough *water* in your body. Being thirsty could be a sign you have lost two per cent of your body water, 11 per cent of your aerobic power, and 45 per cent of your capacity for intense exercise. According to research from University of Aberdeen (UK), water-rich *fruits* and *vegetables* can hydrate your body twice as effectively as a glass of water. Water-rich fruits and vegetables include cucumbers and iceberg lettuce (96 per cent water), tomatoes and apples (94 per cent water), and watermelon and sweet (bell) peppers (92 per cent water).

See *Hydration Percentage*

Dental Hygiene/Dental Care – A research team from the University of Adelaide (Australia) looking at fossilised dental plaque from prehistoric humans found that they had much healthier teeth and gums than we do today. The researchers also compared farmers from the Neolithic era through to modern day humans and found that tooth decay increased with the introduction of farming. It happened again after the *Industrial Revolution* as the diversity of oral bacteria decreased.

Depression – A serious mood disorder that may repeatedly occur over the course of a lifetime. Some symptoms of depression include sadness, insomnia, trouble concentrating, fatigue, and suicidal thoughts. There is evidence that ingestion of *gluten* may contribute to mood disorders and that eliminating gluten may improve cognitive function. *Alcohol* consumption affects the chemistry of the brain, increasing the risk of depression. According to the Office of National Statistics (UK), nearly a fifth of adults experiences anxiety or depression. The most common reasons cited include financial difficulties, relationship conflicts, and major life traumas. Research suggests that these triggers can lead to *serotonin* suppression. Environmental factors that can help depression include increased exposure to *sunlight* and *exercise*, which raise serotonin and dopamine levels and improve *mood*. See *Happiness*

DHA (Docosahexaenoic Acid) – See *Essential Fatty Acids*

Diabetes, diabetic (Diabetes Mellitus) – A disease in which the body is unable to regulate the glucose in the blood. There are two kinds of diabetes, type I and type II. Type I diabetes, formerly known as *juvenile diabetes*, occurs mostly in children and young adults. In this form of the disease, the body is unable to produce *insulin*. Type II diabetes occurs when the body is unable to use insulin properly to manage *blood sugar* levels. At first the body may produce extra insulin to correct the situation, but over time, the body simply cannot keep up, leading to *insulin resistance*. Type II diabetes can be controlled by diet and *exercise*.

Digital Detox – A period where an individual refrains from using technology such as smartphones, computers, and social networking, providing an opportunity to focus on interaction in the real world.

Diet Drinks – Sodas and other drinks usually marketed as *weight loss* drinks. Diet soda and other artificial diet drinks are not part of the *Paleo diet*. Many diet drinks contain *artificial sweeteners*, colours, preservatives, and *caffeine* and can contribute to gut problems, anxiety, and other issues. In addition, the carbon dioxide in sodas may contribute to bone loss or *osteoporosis*.

Dill – A *herb* that is rich in vitamins *A* and *C*. Aids in digestion and *Sleep*.

Dinner – Dinner on the *Paleo diet* should be a healthy combination of *vegetables* and animal *protein*, with some healthy *fats*. An example of a Paleo dinner is a portion of *grass-fed beef* cooked in *coconut oil* along with a big salad or cooked vegetables and some fruit for dessert.

Dirty Dozen (U.S.) – A list of foods produced by the *EWG* that contains the dirtiest conventionally grown (non-organic) *fruits* and *vegetables* in the United States in terms of pesticide residues. As of 2015 this list includes apples, sweet peppers (bell peppers), celery, cherry tomatoes, cucumbers, grapes, nectarines (imported), peaches, potatoes, snap peas (imported), spinach, and strawberries. Additional dirty foods include hot (chili) peppers, kale, and collard greens (UK: spring/fresh greens). If you eat these foods, aim to eat organic whenever possible. See *Clean Fifteen*

Dirty Dozen (UK) – A list of the twelve worst foods for pesticide residues in the United Kingdom, based on data published for the period 2007–2012 by *PAN UK*. The top twelve foods for the five-year period include apples, bananas, cherries, flour, grapefruit (fresh and tinned), lemons, nectarines, oranges, pears, pineapple, soft citrus, and strawberries. If you eat these foods, aim to eat organic whenever possible.

Diseases of Civilisation – See *Lifestyle Disease*

DOMS (Delayed onset muscle soreness) – A dull, aching pain with tenderness and stiffness in the muscles. DOMS can feel uncomfortable but is a regular occurrence after unaccustomed or strenuous exercise. This can occur between twenty-four and seventy-two hours after activity. Some people rest completely during this phase; however, it is better to perform low-intensity work such as *walking* and maintain activity level to increase blood flow to the muscles. DOMS is necessary for muscle growth and adapting to *exercise*, and is an indication that the body is getting used to previous activity.

Dopamine – See *Neurotransmitters*

Dried Fruit – Fruit that has been dried by natural or mechanical means. Dried fruit should be avoided or consumed in tiny quantities because the *sugar* content can be very high. For example, fresh mango contains 15 per cent total sugar while dried mango has 74 per cent. It is also worth noting that fresh fruit contains up to 80 per cent more nutrients and *antioxidants* than dried fruit.

Dysbacteriosis – See *Dysbiosis*

Dysbiosis – A term for a microbial imbalance in the body where harmful bacteria or *yeasts* overpopulate. Occurring most often in the digestive tract, gut dysbiosis is associated with diseases such as colitis, *cancer*, *irritable bowel syndrome*, fatigue, skin problems, and *obesity*. Dietary strategies to manage and reduce dysbiosis include the addition of foods containing *probiotics* such as *fermented foods* as well as *prebiotic* foods. Reducing gut irritants such as *caffeine* and *alcohol* is also beneficial.

The *Paleo diet* can help cure dysbiosis by avoiding gut-damaging processed and refined foods, such as *gluten* and *dairy*, and encouraging gut-healing foods. Gut-healing foods include foods rich in *omega-3* as well as *leafy vegetables*, healthy *fats*, and *bone broth*. Gut dysbiosis often leads to a situation known as *leaky gut*. Many factors are thought to contribute to dysbiosis, including *antibiotics* and other forms of medication, poor diet, and *stress*.

E

"TRUE ENJOYMENT COMES FROM ACTIVITY OF
THE MIND AND EXERCISE OF THE BODY; THE
TWO ARE EVER UNITED."

—WILHELM VON HUMBOLDT

Eating Out – Eating out on the *Paleo diet* can be difficult and may involve some compromise. Tips include asking if the meat is *grass-fed* or organic, what oils are used for preparation, whether the sauces include flour, and asking for virgin olive oil for *salad dressings*.

Eaton, Boyd – See *History of the Paleo Diet*

Eatwell Plate – A pictorial representation (*http://bit.ly/FE-EatWell*) of what the *FSA* consider a healthy, well-balanced diet. It contains the five following food groups:

1. Plenty of bread, rice, *potatoes*, pasta, and other starchy foods
2. Plenty of *fruits* and *vegetables*—eat at least five portions every day
3. Some milk and *dairy*—aim for low-fat options
4. Some meat, *fish*, *eggs*, beans, and other non-dairy sources of protein
5. A small amount of foods containing fat or sugar

Compare the Eatwell Plate, the *USDA Food Pyramid*, and the *Paleo Food Pyramid* to see their differences.

Eggs – A staple ingredient in Paleo breakfasts. In themselves, eggs make a self-contained, well-balanced meal and are a good source of nutrients, such as vitamins *A*, *D*, *B2* and *B12* and a great source of protein however, it is important to choose the best quality eggs you can. When selecting eggs, the first choice is from *pastured* chickens. The second choice is eggs from organic, free range chickens. Avoid eggs from conventional *factory-raised* or caged poultry sources. Liquidised eggs from a carton are also not a healthy choice since they tend to be highly processed. For many years, the official advice was that we should eat a maximum of three eggs a week for fear that the cholesterol in eggs raised the risk of heart disease. However in 2007, the British Heart Foundation as well as other world and UK health organisations revised their guidance in light of scientific evidence that dietary *cholesterol* in eggs were not a risk factor. The current NHS guidelines state that there is no recommended limit on how many eggs people should eat.

Elimination Diet – A method for identifying health issues related to food, such as *allergies*, sensitivities, and symptoms related to *autoimmune diseases*. Suspect foods are eliminated from the diet for a period of time. If the symptoms disappear, foods are reintroduced—one at a time if more than one food is in question—while monitoring for signs of the symptoms returning. *AIP* is an example of an *elimination diet*. Following the AIP may help those with *autoimmune disorders* to identify foods that are exacerbating their symptoms.

EMR (Electromagnetic Radiation) – A type of low-level radiation emitted by electronic equipment, including cell phones. Some studies have suggested a link between cell phone use and an increased risk of brain cancer. The *World Health Organization* classifies EMR as a possible *carcinogen*. Aim to minimise EMR whenever possible by limiting the use of electronics to when absolutely necessary and switching off devices when not in use.

Endocrine Disrupting Chemicals (EDC) – Chemicals that may interfere with the body's *endocrine system*. Studies have linked EDCs to breast, prostate, and testicular cancers; reduced male and female fertility; birth defects; heart disease; several reproductive health issues;

and *diabetes*, as well as possibly affecting brain development and behaviour in young children.

Endocrine System – The network of hormone-producing glands in the human body. *Hormones* are involved in everything from growth and appetite to fertility and disease-fighting ability.

ENS (Enteric Nervous System) – See *Gut-Brain Axis*

E Numbers – A system of codes used to identify approved food additives in the European Union. E numbers or the additive name must appear on food labels. E numbers can be derived from natural sources or synthetic. For example, E numbers that are colours can be natural in origin such as E100 (*curcumin*) which is extracted from *turmeric* root and labelled as Natural Yellow 3 in the U.S., or artificial, such as E102 (*tartrazine*) which is also known as FD&C Yellow 5 in the U.S. There is limited evidence that artificial colours such as tartrazine can trigger, asthma, skin rashes and blurred vision. They are also linked with hyperactivity in some children.

The numbers E249 through E252 are the E numbers for *nitrites* and *nitrates* used in bacon, ham and other cured meats, to stop bacteria from growing. These preservatives may irritate the digestive system causing stomach pains and vomiting, and trigger intestinal problems.

The numbers, E300 through E321 are the E numbers for *antioxidants*, including *vitamins C* and *E* used to stop food going off or changing colour. Some of these additives may cause problems for those with asthma.

Examples of *sweeteners* include E951 (*aspartame*), E954 (*saccharin*) and E420 (*sorbitol*).

E Number categories:

- Colours - E numbers 100-180
- Preservatives - E numbers 200-285
- Antioxidants - E numbers 300-321
- Sweeteners - E numbers 420-421 and 951-959
- Emulsifiers, Stabilisers and Thickeners - 400-495. (E415 is *xanthan gum*, E421 is *guar gum*)
- E numbers above 500, include flavour enhancers such as *monosodium glutamate* (E621), modified starches, bulking agents, and foaming agents.

The European Food Safety Authority is an independent European agency responsible for assessing and approving additives for use.

Any change you can make by adopting a Paleo diet and eliminating the reliance on processed food, which by its very nature requires lots of additives to give it taste, texture, colour, and prolong shelf-life, is a step in the right direction.

Environmental Working Group (EWG) – An independent, not-for-profit American organisation that specialises in researching toxic chemicals. *http://www.ewg.org/*

EPA (Eicosapentaenoic Acid) – See *Essential Fatty Acids*

Epigenetics – The study of how environmental factors influence gene expression (switching genes on or off) or influencing how much the genes can express themselves. The factors that affect gene expression include the ageing process, environment, diet, *exercise*, and *lifestyle*. Epigenetic changes can affect you later in life and can be passed down from generation to generation. Thus, lifestyle decisions can affect not only your own gene expressions, but those of your children and grandchildren. Diseases such as *cancer* and immune disorders can be linked to epigenetics.

Epsom Salt – See *Magnesium*

Essential Fatty Acids (EFA) – *Polyunsaturated fats* that are essential to the diet, since the body is unable to produce them by itself. EFAs help regulate *metabolism* and prostaglandin (*inflammation*) activity within the cells. Because this occurs at the cellular level, the effects of prostaglandin and deficiencies in these EFAs can lead to ill health. The two main categories of EFAs are omega-3 and omega-6 fatty acids. To promote good health, these fatty acids should be eaten in the required amounts and ratio. Both types of fatty acid are essential. However, there is one crucial difference: omega-6 (such as sunflower oil and other seed oils, pumpkin seeds, and sesame seeds) are pro-inflammatory, and omega-3 (found in *oily fish* such as salmon, *walnuts*, naturally raised chicken eggs, and *grass-fed* meat) is *anti-inflammatory*. Maintaining the correct balance of omega-3 to omega-6 is vital to good human health. Our ancestors' *Paleolithic diet* provided a ratio of 1:1 while the modern *Western diet* is closer to 1:16 (omega-3 to omega-6). Studies have shown that both excessive amounts of omega-6 and an exceptionally high ratio to omega-3 (typical in *Western Pattern Diets*) promote *inflammation* and can contribute to the development of *lifestyle diseases* such as cardiovascular disease, *cancer*, and *autoimmune diseases*. Studies suggest the ideal ratio of omega-3 to omega-6 to be between 1:2 and 1:1, similar to the ancestral profile above.

Examples of omega-3 fatty acids include eicosapentaenoic acid (EPA) and docosahexaenoic acid (DHA). EPA and DHA can be formed in the body from another omega-3 fat known as alpha-linolenic acid (ALA) which is found in foods such as *flaxseeds* and walnuts. However, the conversion of ALA to EPA and DHA can be quite poor, so consuming ALA alone may not provide all the benefits to be had from omega-3 fats.

One of the best dietary sources of omega-3 fatty acids is found in wild-caught *oily fish* and has been shown to reduce the tendency of blood clots, lower triglyceride levels, and raise HDL (good) *cholesterol*, all of which mitigate against risk factors associated with heart disease.

Essential Nutrient – A nutrient that cannot be manufactured in the body. Essential nutrients such as *water*, *fats*, *carbohydrates*, and *proteins* can only be obtained through diet. Some essential nutrients can also be obtained through nutritional *supplements* such as *vitamins* and *minerals*.

Estrogen – See *Oestrogen*

Exercise – The benefits of exercise are well documented and include physical, mental, and psychological benefits. Recent studies demonstrate that *inactivity* is linked to poor health. Activity protects us from depression and a wide array of illnesses, and even boosts memory. Exercise on the *Paleo lifestyle* is geared toward movement that mimics the physical activities of our ancestors to the extent that is possible in the modern world.

The human genome was not framed around enduring, recreational, ultra-endurance marathons or exclusively heavy-lifting an object repeatedly to develop fitness. We thrive on a broad repertoire of activity and intensity. We are designed to be movement generalists, multi-skilled and multi-faceted rather than specialists in one or two areas, and our training should reflect this. The types of exercise for which we are designed to do include a variety of activities performed intermittently, at moderate intensities, for reasonable durations. This variety not only improves our physical capability, but also lowers the occurrence of repetitive stress injury, provides inherent motivation, and increases the likelihood for long-term adherence to exercise.

One possible solution is to get back to basics and reference the movement patterns of our hunter-gatherer ancestors: they were naturally lean and strong based on the activities they had to do daily. The book *Paleo Fitness* covers some of those movement patterns and offers strategies that are better geared to the Paleo lifestyle than some conventional fitness programmes.

A research study published in the *Journal of the American College of Cardiology*, which looked at mortality risks in more than 55,000 adults from ages 19 to 100, found that running for just five minutes a day can reduce the risk of dying prematurely by 30 per cent and of dying from cardiovascular causes by 45 per cent. It also increases life expectancy by three years. Running at a slow pace of six miles per hour (9.6 km/h) was enough when compared with not running at all.

Research shows that moderate levels of physical fitness appear to be a protective factor against premature death. A team from the University of Cambridge has found that out of 9.2 million deaths in Europe in 2008, lack of exercise is estimated to contribute to around 676,000 deaths a year, which is almost double the 337,000 deaths estimated to be caused by obesity.

According to a study in the *Journal of the American Medical Association Oncology* published in March 2015, men with higher fitness levels in midlife have a lower risk of lung and colorectal cancer when older. High fitness levels are associated with a two-thirds reduction in cardiovascular death compared with low fitness levels among men who developed cancer at age 65 years or older. See *Sedentary Behaviour*, *Workout Time*, *HIIT*

Experimentation – See *Biohacking*, *Elimination Diet*, *N=1*, *Quantified Self*

EVOO (Extra Virgin Olive Oil) – See *Olive Oil*

EWG – See *Environmental Working Group*

F

"**E**AT HEALTHILY, SLEEP WELL, BREATHE DEEPLY, AND MOVE HARMONIOUSLY."

—JEAN-PIERRE BARRAL

Factory Farmed, factory farms (CAFO) – A

method of farming which keeps animals densely packed into areas smaller than those used in traditional agriculture. Cattle (for meat and dairy production), chickens (for meat and *eggs*), and even fish can be raised in this way. The aim of factory farming is to produce the highest possible amount of product for the lowest possible price. Factory farms are also known as *CAFOs*. They feed the animals corn or manufactured animal feed, and animal health and safety are usually low priorities. Animals raised in this way produce meat and other products that contain higher amounts of fat with higher ratios of *omega-6* to *omega-3* than is healthy. The preference is to consume naturally reared or *pastured* meats.

Farm to Fork – The UK equivalent of *Farm to Table*, also known as *Field to Fork*.

Farm to Table – A movement in the U.S. concerned with delivering local food to local consumers.

Fasting Glucose – A measurement of *blood sugar* performed after a fast of at least eight hours. It is usually part of regular *blood work*.

Fat Loss – A reduction in overall body fat as a percentage of total body composition. Fat loss is calculated as a reduction percentage. For example, a reduction of body fat from 25 per cent to 20 per cent is presented as five per cent total fat loss. Fat loss can lead to *weight loss*, but this is not guaranteed, as lean body mass is denser than fat. You may weigh more but be smaller in size due to increased lean body mass and reduced body fat.

Fats – A family of compounds called lipids that are essential for health and are critical components of diet. The role of dietary fats is open to considerable debate, but the importance of fats in human physiology should not be underestimated. Fats are part of the structural components of the membranes around every cell in the body; they constitute the majority of the structure of the brain (around 60%), central nervous system, and spinal cord; maintain the health of blood vessels; are involved in the process of making steroid **hormones** such as **testosterone**; aid in the regulation of enzymes; provide insulation through **adipose tissue** just under the skin and store energy there; transport, store, and utilise the **fat-soluble vitamins A, D, E**, and **K**; are a high-octane fuel source; and control **inflammation**. Low levels of dietary fat have been linked to memory and learning deficiencies, infertility, increased risk of **depression**, and age-related conditions such as Parkinson's, Alzheimer's, and arthritis.

There are three core types of fats: saturated, monounsaturated, and polyunsaturated. Saturated fats come from foods such as **eggs** and meats. See **History of Fat** to see why saturated fat is no longer demonised as it once was. **Monounsaturated fats** are found in sources such as avocados and olives, and polyunsaturated fats are found in **fish, nuts**, and **seeds**.

See **Carbohydrates, Protein**

Fat-Soluble Vitamins – Vitamins that are found mainly in animal fats, liver, and **oily fish**. They are stored by the body for future use and can be harmful if much more is stored than is needed. If you are taking fat-soluble vitamins in *supplement* form, take them with meals containing fat to aid absorption. Vitamins *A*, *D*, *E*, and *K* are fat soluble. See *Water-Soluble Vitamins*

FDA (Food and Drug Administration) – A U.S. federal agency that falls under the Department of Health and Human Services. The FDA is responsible for food safety and regulation as well as drug testing and approval, including regulating over-the-counter medicines and nutritional *supplements*. The FDA also monitors animal feed and veterinary practices.
See *USDA*

Fermentation (Ferment) – A process that converts *sugar* into alcohol, acid, or gas. Humans have enjoyed *fermented foods* and drink since the *Neolithic Age*. See *Alcohol*

Fermented Foods – Foods that undergo the process of fermentation such as sauerkraut, kimchee, and *kombucha*. Fermented foods can be a great source of *probiotics*.
See *Prebiotics*

Fibromyalgia – A chronic condition that causes muscle pain all over the body. Fibromyalgia affects seven times more women than men.

Fibre – Dietary fibre is a complex carbohydrate which cannot be digested by the human body and passes through our digestive system. There are two primary types of fibre, soluble (fruit, vegetables) and insoluble (whole grains, nuts, seeds and fruit peel). The Paleo diet is a great source of fibre, with options including, sweet potatoes, beetroots and other root vegetables, leafy green vegetables, and fruits such as apples, pears, and berries. Excess insoluble fibre can bind to *minerals* such as zinc, magnesium, and iron and block absorption of these nutrients.

Fight-Or-Flight – See *Sympathetic Nervous System*

Fish – An excellent Paleo food. Aim for wild-caught, sustainable fish such as salmon, haddock, sardines, cod, mackerel, and trout. Farmed variants are less nutritious.

Fish Oil – Supplements that contain *omega-3* fatty acids, including *EPA* and *DHA*. Some studies have found that evidence for the benefits of taking supplemental fish oil is limited. However, the bulk of evidence points to heart-health benefits. For example, one gram of fish oil can cut the risk of death by heart attack by as much as 20 per cent.

Fitness – A measure of human health, particularly of the *strength*, endurance, and *flexibility* of the body.

Five-a-Day Campaign (UK) – A campaign launched by the UK's Department of Health. The Five-a-Day Campaign is based on a recommendation in 1990 from the *World Health Organization* to eat at least five portions of *fruits* and *vegetables* every day to prevent chronic disease. A serving is 80g (2.8oz). From a Paleo perspective, most portions should comprise vegetables, with infrequent fruit consumption.

Flaxseeds – Tiny seeds that contain *omega-3* and *omega-6 essential fatty acids* as well as *vitamin E*, *vitamin B3*, and a wide variety of *minerals*. Flaxseeds should be stored in a cool, dry place. They best consumed by either soaking them overnight in water or grinding them into a meal just prior to consumption.

Flaxseeds are *prebiotics*, which help promote the growth of *probiotics*, the good bacteria in the gut. They have wide-ranging health benefits, including aiding digestion. Recent studies have shown that the compounds (*lignans*) in flaxseeds may:

- help protect against several forms of cancer, including breast and colon cancer
- help prevent atherosclerosis in heart disease
- improve *blood glucose balance* in *diabetics*
- reduce hot flushes in menopause

There are two main varieties of flaxseed: brown and yellow/golden (golden linseed).

Flexitarians – Semi-*vegetarians* who occasionally consume fish, meat, and poultry.

Flexibility – Refers to the optimal range of movement in the muscle and joints to allow bending and motion. Overall flexibility should be adequate to meet the physical demands placed on the body that typically means a normal range of motion is sufficient for most activities. Stretching is often used to improve flexibility, however stretching for too long or too often increases the likelihood of injury. See *Sarcopenia, Balance, Strength*

F.lux *http://justgetflux.com/* – Free software used to minimise the risk of disrupting your *sleep cycle* by adjusting the computer display automatically based on location and the time of day. See *Sleep Tips*

FODMAP – An acronym for *fermentable oligo-, di-, monosaccharides and polyols.* Examples of FODMAPs are *wheat*, barley, rye, onions, cabbage, broccoli, and pistachio nuts. Some people consume too many FODMAPs for the body to absorb. When this happens, the FODMAPs pass from the small intestine to the large intestine, where bacteria cause them to ferment. This can lead to bloating, gas, stomach cramps, and *IBS.*

Following a *low-FODMAP diet* can help to alleviate or eliminate these symptoms. Studies show that FODMAP foods absorb more water, which speeds up gut transit time and increases the risk of diarrhoea.

Folate – See *Vitamin B9*

Folic Acid – See *Vitamin B9*

Food Allergy – An adverse physical reaction to a specific food or foods. With a true food allergy, the body produces elevated levels of *immunoglobulin* E (IgE) and subsequently *histamine* in response to ingestion of a specific food. This is the same immunoglobulin which becomes active in non-food *allergies* such as hay fever and dust mites. Typically, a reaction, often coughing or sneezing, occurs immediately after exposure but the onset of symptoms can be minutes to hours after exposure. Severe reactions may result in swelling in the mouth and throat, causing breathing problems and other issues that can become life threatening. Doctors can perform tests for IgE reactions, which may involve a blood, scratch or skin/patch test. Up to 90 per cent of food allergies are triggered by the *Big 8 foods*.

Food Consumption – Humans have a biological drive to seek out high-calorie foods in time of plenty to ensure survival once foods become scarce. Nowadays, we are consuming more food (whether healthy or not) at relatively lower cost than ever before but without the periods of scarcity, which leads to over-consumption. For example, the average American ate 23 per cent less food in 1970 than in 2010. In 1950, the largest serving of a typical soft drink was eight ounces (227ml). In 2015, a small serving is 16 ounces (455ml) and the double gulp is 64 ounces (1.89 litres), containing nearly fifty teaspoons of *sugar.* The average restaurant meal today is more than four times larger than in the 1950s. The surface area of the average dinner plate at home has increased 36 per cent since 1960. Research by the British Heart Foundation found that in the last 20 years, individual pie sizes grew by 40 per cent and ready meals by 50 per cent.

Food Intolerance – A reaction to a food, beverage, or additive. Food intolerance is also known as *non-allergic food hypersensitivity.* It may involve immunoglobulins such as IgG (but not IgE) or enzyme deficiencies such those found in *lactose intolerance.* Diagnosis is more difficult to ascertain than with a *food allergy* because the reaction is often delayed. While the result is detrimental and ranges from respiratory and skin problems (rashes, dermatitis) to digestion problems, it is not an actual allergic reaction because the body does not produce **antibodies** to the food in question. Some food intolerances are thought to be due to a condition known as *leaky gut.* If you suspect a food intolerance, try experimenting with an *elimination diet.* Food intolerances can be a contributing factor in *autoimmune disorders.*

Food Quantity – See *Food Consumption*

Food Standards Agency (FSA) – A UK government agency responsible for public health in relation to food.

Food Storage – See *Utensils*

Foraging – The art of searching for and obtaining wild foods.

Free-Range – A term that describes both a method of raising livestock (in which animals are free to roam outdoors rather than being in indoor enclosures; (see *Factory Farmed*) and the *meat, eggs,* and other products that are derived from animals raised in this manner. While free-range animals may be indoors for part of the time, when they are outside they get sunlight and may eat what they choose, including the grasses and insects that are part of their natural diet. The term *free-range* may apply to cattle, chicken, and other livestock. See *Organic*

Fructose – The type of *sugar* found in *fruits*. The body absorbs fructose directly into the bloodstream during digestion, so consumption of high amounts of fructose may contribute to *high blood sugar*, *diabetes* and fatty liver disease. The foods with the highest levels of fructose are refined sweeteners such as high-fructose corn syrup (HFCS), also called corn sugar, and sweeteners such as honey, agave nectar, and maple syrup, as well as *fruits* and fruit juices.

Fruit – An important part of the *Paleo diet*. Most of the carbohydrates in the Paleo diet should come from *fruits* and *vegetables*. Fruit does contain high amounts of *fructose*, so limit fruit intake to one or two pieces a day. For *weight loss*, avoid high-fructose options such as bananas and grapes. Fruit examples include apples, apricots, avocados, berries, citrus fruits, dates, grapes, kiwi fruit, melons, peaches, and pears.

Fruit Juice – The juice that is extracted from *fruits*. Drinking fruit juices unnecessarily increases the *insulin* load because of the removal of the fibrous part of the fruit. It is unlikely that you would eat eight whole oranges, but you could easily consume the juice from eight oranges in a few seconds. The attending high *sugar* content negates the health benefits of the juice. Just eat the whole fruit instead. See *Smoothies, Juicing*

G

"THE GOAL OF LIFE IS TO MAKE YOUR
HEARTBEAT MATCH THE BEAT OF THE UNIVERSE,
TO MATCH YOUR NATURE WITH NATURE."

—JOSEPH CAMPBELL

Game – The term for any undomesticated or wild animal that is hunted for food. Game meat is typically leaner than farmed meat. Some common types of game meat are venison (deer), rabbit, bison, bear, wild boar, and wild-caught fish.

GAPS Diet (Gut and Psychology Syndrome) – A diet developed by Dr Natasha Campbell-McBride, a neurologist and nutritionist who works in the treatment of autism, schizophrenia, ADD/ADHD, and other problems. She developed the GAPS diet to treat the gut imbalance that is at the core of many of these illnesses. The GAPS diet typically begins with an intense detoxification period, during which the patient eats an extremely limited diet of easily digested meats, *vegetables*, and *broth*. After the detox period, those following the GAPS diet may add other foods; however, *grains*, *sugars*, and *tubers* are still avoided. Parents of children with autism report that their children have become more communicative and expressive of emotion after following the GAPS diet; others following the diet have experienced relief of their gastrointestinal symptoms.

Garlic – Garlic is a member of the same family as onions and leaks. Garlic contains vitamin C, vitamin B6, sulphur, *selenium*, and antioxidants. There is some evidence that garlic can reduce infections, lower *blood pressure*, and offer protection against cancer of the digestive tract.

Gastrointestinal (GI) Tract – See *Gut*

Gedgaudas, Nora – Author of the book, *Primal Body, Primal Mind: Beyond the Paleo Diet for Total Health and A Longer Life.* Nora is a speaker and educator on the Paleo diet.

Gelatine (or Gelatin) – A colourless, flavourless, clear food product made from the connective tissue of animals. Obtain gelatine from *pastured* or wild-caught sources, or make your own by making *bone broth.* Benefits include improved digestion, gut health, skin, hair, nails, and joint repair.

Genetic Testing – A DNA test that looks for changes in a person's genes or chromosomes. Genetic testing can reveal hereditary conditions such as sickle-cell anaemia, determine genetic risk factors for diseases such as Parkinson's, and even show physical traits such as hair colour and pain threshold levels. It can determine a person's ancestry and even how closely related an individual is to Neanderthals.

Genetic tests are performed using genotype technology to analyse the DNA in a saliva sample. The testing company 23andMe offers ancestry information and the raw genetic information without interpretation in the United States. In the United Kingdom and Canada, the company currently reports on more than 240 health conditions and traits.

GERD (Gastrointestinal Esophageal Reflux Disease) – See *Acid Reflux*

Ghee – A dairy product made from cow or buffalo milk by simmering butter and milk solids, then evaporating the water until it caramelises, leaving behind golden butterfat. Ghee is nearly 100 per cent fat; thus, all the carbohydrates such as lactose have been removed, and only the smallest traces of milk protein such as *casein* remain. Ghee can be used as a cooking fat - obtain from quality sources.

Ghrelin – An enzyme produced in the stomach, also known as the *hunger hormone*. When the stomach is empty, the ghrelin cells secrete ghrelin, signalling the body that it is time to eat. Ghrelin also helps the body regulate the release of energy, stimulates the release of *growth hormone* and plays a role in regulating addictions and sexual desire. When the stomach is full, the body stops releasing ghrelin. See *Leptin, Sleep*

Ginger – A *spice* with *anti-inflammatory* properties. Ginger can promote healthy digestion and prevent nausea. Make your own fresh ginger tea by steeping a cube of fresh ginger in hot water and adding a slice of lemon and some fresh *mint.*

GI (Gastrointestinal) Tract – See *Gut*

Glucagon – A hormone that performs the opposite function of *insulin.* Glucagon increases the level of glucose in the bloodstream when levels are very low.

Gluconeogenesis – A metabolic function that produces glucose from non-carbohydrates in order to prevent hypoglycaemia or low **blood sugar**.

Glucose – A simple **sugar** (monosaccharide) found in plants. It is one of three sugars (along with dextrose and galactose) that is absorbed directly into the blood stream during digestion. The body uses glucose as a source of fuel. However, having too high a level of glucose in the blood is dangerous. Doctors use a **fasting blood test** to check glucose levels. A high fasting glucose level may signal either pre-diabetes or **diabetes**.

Glutamine (also known as *L-glutamine*) – An amino acid the body uses for several essential functions, including protein synthesis, regulation of acid in the kidneys, and transport of ammonium through the bloodstream. Glutamine also aids in the healing process. Some dietary sources of glutamine include chicken, fish, beef, eggs, and **vegetables** such as cabbage, spinach, beets, and parsley.

Gluten – A protein comprising glutenin and gliadin found in **grains**, including **wheat**, oats, barley, and rye. Gluten is the component that allows baked goods to maintain their form and avoid crumbling apart. While grains are the best-known sources of gluten, many other food products contain gluten as well, including sauces and beers. It is also an additive in everything from ice cream to condiments.

The **Paleo diet** eliminates grains and other sources of gluten. Gluten is hard to digest, blocks absorption of vitamins and alters good gut bacteria, leading to an increased risk of **yeast** and bacterial infections. It may cause **leaky gut syndrome** and be a contributing factor in many **autoimmune diseases**, most notably **coeliac disease**. The books *Grain Brain* by David Perlmutter and *Wheat Belly* by William Davis offer interesting insights into the issues with gluten.

Gluten Free – A product that is free from **gluten**. Be aware that there are many gluten-free products that are full of artificial additives, poor quality fats, and lots of sugar, or are made from non-glutenous grains. Gluten-free products can still contain trace elements of gluten which can be an issue for those suffering from **coeliac disease**.

Gluten Sensitivity – See *Non-Coeliac Gluten Sensitivity*

Glycaemic Index (U.S. Glycemic Index) – A system also known as *GI* that measures how quickly and how high *blood sugar* levels rise after a given food. Most foods have numbers between 50 and 100, although the scale ranges from 1 to 100. The glycaemic index categorises foods as high GI (above 85), moderate GI (60-85), low GI (below 60). Glycaemic responses may vary from person to person based on overall health. A person with *diabetes*, for example, might have elevated glucose levels for hours after eating something with a high glycaemic index number, while a person with normal blood sugar might return to normal very quickly. See *Glycaemic Load*

Glycaemic Load (U.S. Glycemic Load) – A system also referred to as *GL* that describes the quality (*glycaemic index*) value but also takes into account the quantity of carbohydrate that is contained within the food. The glycaemic load is calculated by multiplying the glycaemic index by the amount of carbohydrate in grams and dividing the total by 100.

The GL is categorised as:

- high (above 20)
- moderate (11-19)
- low (10 or below)

For example, a bagel and watermelon both have a GI of 72, however the bagel has a GL of 25 and the watermelon a GL of four. There is over six times the carb load in the bagel. The bagel will require much more of an insulin response than the watermelon. After a low GL meal, blood sugar and insulin levels rise less, there is increased satiety (*feeling full*), delayed hunger, and decreased subsequent food intake in comparison to high GL meals.

Glycogen – A form of glucose stored in the liver and muscle tissue for future use. In the event of a glucose shortage, the liver or muscles convert glycogen back into glucose.

GM (Genetically Modified) – See **GMO**

GMO (Genetically Modified Organism) – Any organism that scientists have genetically engineered to be different from its original state. While humans have cross-bred plants and animals for centuries to ensure hardier specimens, recent scientific developments in biotechnology now allow scientists to rapidly isolate, add, and remove individual genes and insert them into the DNA of a plant or animal that does not naturally produce this protein. For example, ***Big Agra*** companies genetically modify crops to make them resistant to pests and herbicides or to ensure higher crop yields. Some hazards of GMOs include gut and digestive problems, ***autoimmune diseases***, and damage to the environment.

Goitre – The name of a swelling at the front of the neck, an enlargement of the thyroid gland caused by ***iodine deficiency***. A goitre is the most obvious sign of deficiency because the thyroid gland's job is to produce the thyroid hormone, which it does using iodine. If the body isn't getting enough iodine, the gland expands to try to produce more on its own.

Goitrogen – A type of *antinutrient* that depresses thyroid function. It is found in the class of plants called '*brassica*', such as Brussels sprouts, broccoli, kale, and cabbage. It is also found in Soya. *Cooking* removes most of the goitrogens in these foods.

GORD (Gastro-Oesophageal Reflux Disease) – See *Acid Reflux*

Grain-Fed – The term for animals fattened on corn, *soya*, and similar types of feed. Grains comprise the majority of the diet typically used to fatten these animals. Feeding them grains also increases yield and decreases fattening time and the quantity of *omega-3* fats.

Grain-Finished – The term for *grass-fed* animals that are fattened on corn, *soya*, and other types of feed for the last few months before slaughter.

Grains – A family of foods that include *wheat*, oats, rye, barley, amaranth, millet, and rice. Prior to the *Neolithic Revolution*, grains were not part of the human diet because humans did not yet cultivate food. Grains are now a significant part of many people's diet, but they can be harmful for various reasons. Poor grain storage may cause contamination with **aflatoxins**. Grains can also be difficult to digest and may contribute to *leaky gut syndrome* and *autoimmune disorders*. *Soaking* grains can reduce, but not eliminate, the risk of antinutrients. Grains offer no nutrients we cannot obtain from plant and animal foods. A study published in *Nutrition Research* (May 2015) tested a grain-free Paleo diet against a grain-based heart-healthy diet as recommended by the American Heart Association. The Paleo diet improved heart health and induced weight loss significantly more than the conventional dietary recommendations based on a four-month comparison.

Grass-Fed – Animals that are fed only or mostly grass. Grass comprises the majority of the diet for grass-fed cattle, which improves the nutritional quality of the *meat*. For example, all beef contains *omega-3* fats, but grass-fed beef has up to three times more than *grain-fed* meat. See *Pastured*

Grass-Finished – A term typically used to describe grass-fed animals that are not butchered during the growth stage and fed grass until physical maturity.

Graves' Disease – See *Hyperthyroidism*

Green Revolution – An attempt by agroecologists and other scientists to steer agriculture away from reliance on fossil fuels and toward a more sustainable model that will feed more people while also protecting the earth. The goal is to improve soil quality by reducing the use of pesticides, reducing waste by recycling biological materials, and improving crop yields by introducing biodiversity and reducing the effects of solar radiation and erosion.

Green Tea – See *Tea*

Growth Hormone – Steroid hormones used to make animals gain weight faster and to ensure less food is used before an animal is slaughtered. In dairy cows, growth hormones can also be used to increase milk production. Products from hormone-treated animals should be avoided, as residues of these hormones can remain in meat and milk with potential harmful health effects. In 1989, the European Union banned the use of growth hormone on all meat from animals and dairy cattle. See **Human Growth Hormone**

Guar Gum (E421) – A product from the seeds of plants that belong to the pea family. Food manufacturers use guar gum as a thickener, preservative, and emulsifier. You may need to avoid this product if you follow a **low-FODMAP diet**. See **E Numbers**

Gut – The gastrointestinal tract. The term '*gut*' usually specifically refers to the stomach and intestines. See **Gut Flora, Gut-Brain Axis**

Gut-Brain Axis – The term for a complex communications system between the **gut flora** and the brain. There is evidence to suggest that gut flora may play a role in brain function. We often associate **hormones** such as **serotonin** with the brain, but more than 95 per cent of serotonin resides in the gut. This underscores the importance of maintaining a healthy balance of gut flora, as that balance may affect brain function.

Gut Flora – Micro-organisms that live in the intestines and also known as *gut microbiota.* Gut flora ferments undigested carbohydrates and converts them to energy. Imbalances or *dysbiosis*, in the gut flora, can lead to *leaky gut*, a compromised *immune system*, and *obesity.* See *Microbiome*

Gut Microbiome – See *Gut Flora*

Gut Permeability – See *Leaky Gut Syndrome*

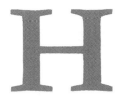

"PHYSICAL FITNESS IS NOT ONLY ONE OF THE
MOST IMPORTANT KEYS TO A HEALTHY BODY; IT
IS THE BASIS OF DYNAMIC AND CREATIVE
INTELLECTUAL ACTIVITY."

—JOHN F. KENNEDY

Haemoglobin – The protein that transports oxygen in the blood. See **Iron**

Happiness – Having a more altruistic outlook on life is beneficial, since happiness that comes from having a deep sense of purpose has been shown to reduce inflammation. See **Depression**

Hashimoto's thyroiditis – See **Hypothyroidism**

HbA1c (Haemoglobin A1c) – A kind of **haemoglobin** used to measure the glucose concentration in blood plasma. It is also known as *glycated haemoglobin* or *glycosylated haemoglobin*. High levels of HbA1c are linked to many diseases. The test for HbA1c provides information on average blood sugar levels over a two- to three-month period before the test. See **Blood Work**

HDL (High-Density Cholesterol) – See **Cholesterol**

HEALTH *Unplugged* – The first European Paleo conference ever held HEALTH Unplugged focussed on health and well-being through ancestral nutrition, fitness, and lifestyle. Founded by Darryl Edwards. The inaugural event took place in London, UK on 25 October 2014. More details at *http://www.healthunplugged.co.uk*.

Heavy Metals – A range of toxic metals that includes *lead*, *mercury*, and *cadmium*.

Hemoglobin – See *Haemoglobin*

Herbs (See *Spices and Herbs*) – Use herbs and spices as a substitute for salt.

High Blood Pressure – See *Hypertension*

HIIT (High-Intensity Interval Training) – A form of *exercise* that alternates short periods of very intense anaerobic exercise with recovery periods. It can be helpful in boosting *metabolism*, improving muscle tone and burning fat. A popular form of interval training is based on the *Tabata* protocol. According to a 2011 study presented at the American College of Sports Medicine (ACSM), just 2 weeks of high-intensity intervals improves your aerobic capacity as much as 6 to 8 weeks of endurance training. The benefits of HIIT include improvements in:

- aerobic and anaerobic fitness
- blood pressure
- cardiovascular health
- insulin sensitivity
- cholesterol profile
- body composition

See *Sprinting*

Histamine – A compound released by cells in response to allergic and inflammatory reactions, which causes local swelling, redness and itching.

History of Fat – For years we have been *'fed'* the simple message, *Eat fat—get fat*. The following is some history of concerns about fat and the current views on fat.

- 1958 – The physiologist Ancel Keys starts his *Seven Countries Study*, which showed saturated fat as a root cause of heart disease. (Much later, it was discovered that his results were cherry-picked to support his hypothesis; he had dismissed the fifteen countries that showed no association).
- 1961 – Keys appears on the cover of *Time Magazine* and is on the committee of the American Heart Association, which advises Americans to cut back on saturated fat for the first time.
- 1970 – The Keys study is published amidst massive media interest.

- 1972 – *Dr. Atkins' Diet Revolution* and *Pure, White and Deadly* are published.
- 1980 – "Dietary Guidelines for Americans", is published, based on U.S. Senator George McGovern's 1977 report. It advises eating more starches and reducing dietary fat intake.
- 1984 – *Time Magazine*: The front cover depicts cholesterol as the bad guy, with an accompanying article entitled 'Hold the eggs and butter', about the most expensive research project in medical history.
- 1984 – UK government adopts lowering saturated fat and advises people to get no more than 10 per cent of their calories from saturated fat.
- 2009 – Dr Robert Lustig's lecture "Sugar: The Bitter Truth" prompts an anti-sugar crusade.
- 2013 – After a two-year study, the Swedish government recommends a low-carb/high-fat diet.
- 2013 – *The Real Meal Revolution* is published, with the author Professor Tim Noakes denouncing his previously held views on a high carbohydrate diet and switching to a low-carb, high-fat diet.
- 2014 – A meta-analysis published in *Annals of Internal Medicine* concludes that evidence does not support the idea that diets low in saturated fat are healthy.
- 2014 – *Time Magazine's* "Eat Butter" cover is published. In the United Kingdom, the NHS website states, "Researchers say they have found no significant link between saturated fat and heart disease." However, the current guidelines remain unchanged.

History of the Paleo Diet – Many assume the Paleo diet is a new way of eating; however, the idea of discussing the merits of ancestral foods versus modern foods has been around for over one hundred years. Let's take a look at some of the Paleo family tree.

Great-grandparents – The discussion arguably begins with a book published in 1913 by Vilhjalmur Stefansson called *My Life with the Eskimo*, based on the explorer's experience living with the Inuits and consuming their traditional diet, which consisted mainly of animal fats and protein with very little carbohydrates.

In 1939, a book by **Dr Weston A. Price** was published, entitled *Nutrition and Physical Degeneration: A Comparison of Primitive and Modern Diets and Their Effects*. Dr Price is the great-grandfather of the Paleo movement. He travelled extensively across the globe for a more than a decade to study isolated and non-Westernised populations, making observations about their diet, health, and lifestyle in comparison to the American diet of the time. He concluded that whenever the non-Westernised people's traditional diets were replaced with modern convenience foods, their health and physical state suffered.

Grandparents – In 1975 gastroenterologist Dr Walter Voegtlin published a book called *The Stone Age Diet: Based on In-depth Studies of Human Ecology and the Diet of Man*. This book documented how Dr Voegtlin treated patients with severe digestive disorders such as **Crohn's disease** with a diet replicating the eating habits of Paleolithic humans. A decade later, a research paper was published in the *New England Journal of Medicine* entitled *Paleolithic nutrition: A consideration of its nature and current implications* by Boyd Eaton and Melvin Konner. They took the Paleolithic premise further and backed up Dr Voegtlin's ideas. The popularity and acceptance of their ideas by the mainstream medical establishment led to the late-1980s book *The Paleolithic Prescription* by Eaton, Konner, and Marjorie Shostak.

Parents – In the 1990s, Swedish medical doctor and scientist **Staffan Lindeberg** published "The Kitava Study" based on the findings of his work with present-day **hunter-gatherers** in Papua New Guinea. His research established that their traditional diet helped prevent stroke, ischemic heart disease, *diabetes*, *obesity*, and *hypertension*.

In 1995, Ray Audette wrote the book *NeanderThin: A Caveman's Guide to Nutrition* after he successfully treated his *rheumatoid arthritis* and *type II diabetes* with diet. His research stemmed from the notion that what humans ate before agriculture and technology is what we need today to be healthy and lean and stave off disease. The book was republished in 2000 as *NeanderThin: Eat Like a Caveman to Achieve a Lean, Strong, Healthy Body*.

Nutrition and fitness expert *Loren Cordain*'s research led to the 2002 publication of his book *The Paleo Diet: Lose Weight and Get Healthy by Eating the Food You Were Designed to Eat*. This book looked at the anthropological evidence behind the health changes that occurred after humans adopted an agriculture-based diet and lifestyle. Dr Cordain also points out the fundamental concepts that modern humans differ genetically from our *hunter-gatherer* ancestors by a mere 0.02 per cent and that this genetic heritage is largely discordant with life today.

Sons and Daughters – In the last few years many people have endorsed the lifestyle and teachings of the concepts described above, including the authors of bestselling books such as *The Paleo Solution* (**Robb Wolf**), *The Primal Blueprint* (**Mark Sisson**), and *Practical Paleo* (Diane Sanfilippo). These experts have taken the essence of this message and spread the good news to the masses, with the result of bringing the healthy choice of a *Paleo lifestyle* to millions.

The Extended Family – Currently in the Paleo community there is much debate about what does and does not constitute Paleo. For example, debates are raging on the proportion of carbohydrates that should be eaten, whether *dairy* is safe to consume, and whether drinking high-fat coffee is the best way to start the day. However, there are seven fundamental concepts that are important to focus on, and on which most Paleo proponents agree:

1. Be omnivorous—eat both animals and plants.
2. Use traditional food preparation techniques.
3. Draw inspiration from our ancestors' dietary patterns.
4. Eat fresh, whole, and preferably local, unprocessed foods of the highest nutrient quality.
5. Avoid industrialised, processed, and artificial foods.

6. Avoid *toxins* and *antinutrients* that impede digestion.
7. Know the source of your food.

Hormones – Chemicals secreted by several types of glands. Hormones are messengers that flow around the body, travelling through the bloodstream. They influence who you are—both mentally and physically—and regulate functions such as reproduction, *metabolism*, disease resistance, digestion, *sleep*, growth, immune responses, and *mood*. Hormone imbalances can cause a variety of health issues, including weight gain, *acne*, fatigue, *diabetes*, *sleep disruption*, and mood swings. Many things may contribute to a hormone imbalance, such as poor nutrition, *jetlag*, and *chronic stress*.

Human Growth Hormone (HGH) – A hormone that stimulates growth in children, repair and rejuvenation in adults, is a potent anti-ageing agent and plays a role in a healthy *metabolism*. We make most of our growth hormone at night during deep sleep (the most restorative stage of the *sleep cycle*) from the pituitary gland at the base of the brain. Insufficient growth hormone in adults is associated with fat accumulating around the middle and premature ageing.

Hunter-Gatherer – A person who finds food by hunting, fishing, and foraging rather than cultivating. Our Paleolithic ancestors were hunter-gatherers. They ate animals they killed and plants they gathered from their surroundings. The hunter-gatherer diet is the basis of the *Paleo diet*.

Hydration Percentage – This is the level of *water* in the body expressed as a percentage of total weight. Your body water levels naturally fluctuate throughout the day and night. Your body tends to be *dehydrated* after a long night, and there are differences in fluid distribution between day and night. Eating large meals, drinking alcohol, menstruation, illness, exercising, and bathing may cause variations in your hydration levels. Finding the right balance of water intake will ensure that your body functions efficiently, helping you to stay healthy. See *Dehydration*

Hydrochloric Acid (HCl) – See *Acid Reflux*

Hydrogenated Fats – See *Trans Fats*

Hygiene Hypothesis – A medical theory that children who are not exposed to bacteria (including gut flora or *probiotics*), dirt and other *pathogens* early in life may have a higher chance of developing *allergies* and *autoimmune disorders*. After the *industrial revolution*, there were a number of ways in which people fought childhood infections, including pasteurization, sterilization, and vaccination. The hygiene hypothesis states that our *immune systems* may not develop properly if our bodies are not exposed to the things they need to fight. See *Leaky Gut Syndrome*

Hypertension (High Blood Pressure) – The term for abnormally high *blood pressure*. Chronic hypertension is known as the world's biggest '*silent killer*', as it has no visible signs or symptoms. It is one of the most common causes of premature death and disability, as it can lead to strokes and heart and kidney failure. In 2012, the British medical journal *The Lancet* published large-scale research that identified hypertension as the world's biggest killer.

Physical activity (sedentary people have a 35 per cent greater risk of developing high blood pressure) and a reduction of **stress** can help to lower blood pressure, while **smoking**, **alcohol**, **caffeine**, and other foods can increase blood pressure. Foods that can help lower blood pressure include watermelon, which contains L-citrulline, an amino acid that has been shown to lower blood pressure, and **garlic**, which contains allicin a compound that is released when garlic is crushed; it works on the kidneys to help lower blood pressure. Inorganic nitrates from root vegetables such as beetroot have also been shown to cause a long-lasting reduction in blood pressure in individuals with hypertension; inorganic nitrate is converted into nitric oxide in the body, which then relaxes and dilates blood vessels. Leafy green vegetables such as lettuce and cabbage also contain inorganic nitrate. It is also recommended to reduce salt intake by avoiding processed, convenience, and artificial foods. See **Hypotension**

Hyperthyroidism – The term for an overactive thyroid, which is when the thyroid gland produces too much thyroid hormone. The exact cause is unknown however it is believed to be a combination of genetic and environmental factors. The most common cause of hyperthyroidism is *Graves' disease* which is an **autoimmune disease** that affects the thyroid. See **Hypothyroidism**

Hypotension (Low Blood Pressure) – The term for abnormally low **blood pressure**. Usually, low blood pressure is nothing to worry about, however if your blood pressure drops too low it can restrict blood flow to the brain which can lead to light-headiness or fainting. See **Hypertension**

Hypothyroidism – The term for underactive thyroid, which is when the thyroid gland does not produce enough thyroid hormone. The two leading causes of hypothyroidism are insufficient iodine in the diet or the **autoimmune disease** Hashimoto's thyroiditis in which the thyroid gland is attacked by the **immune system**. There is evidence that Selenium deficiency may be a causative factor in hypothyroidism. See **Hyperthyroidism**

I

"THE FOOD YOU EAT CAN EITHER BE THE
SAFEST AND MOST POWERFUL FORM OF
MEDICINE OR THE SLOWEST FORM OF POISON."

—ANN WIGMORE

IBS (Irritable Bowel Syndrome) – A disease of the gastrointestinal system characterized by pain, bloating, gas, and bowel disruption. *Stress* and diet may contribute to IBS, and following the *Paleo diet* may help to relieve its symptoms and even prevent its occurrence. Be aware that other diseases of the gastrointestinal system have symptoms similar to IBS, such as *coeliac disease* and certain parasitic infections.

Immune Response – A reaction of the body to help it fight infection and recover from injury. See *Immune System*

Immune System – A biological system that helps an organism ward off disease and infection. In order to function properly, the immune system must be able to identify any potential risk to the body, including foreign invaders such as *pathogens* correctly. When the body's immune system is not as active as it should be, an immunodeficiency can result. For example, acquired diseases such as HIV/AIDS, genetic disease, and taking immunosuppressive medications can all result in immunodeficiency.

When the immune system fails to distinguish between healthy tissue and *antigens*, the result is an *autoimmune disease*. This means that the body's immune system is attacking healthy tissue rather than antigens. The *Paleo diet*, especially the autoimmune protocol (*AIP*) can help to diminish or even eliminate the symptoms of many autoimmune diseases.

Immunoglobulin (Antibodies) – Proteins that are produced by the *immune system* to help get rid of *antigens*.

Inactivity – See *Sedentary Behaviour, Exercise*

Increased Intestinal Permeability – See *Leaky Gut Syndrome*

Indigestion – Any condition of disrupted or upset digestion. Symptoms of indigestion include gas and abdominal pain. *Acid reflux* may sometimes cause indigestion. It may also be a symptom of a more serious problem, such as ulcerative disease or cancer. While it is difficult to attribute most indigestion to a specific cause, some contributing factors may be underlying disease, diet, or drugs such as **NSAIDs** (non-steroidal anti-inflammatories).

Industrial Revolution – The period of time starting in 1760 and ending between 1820 and 1840. During this period, technological advancements led to sweeping changes in manufacturing. Prior to the Industrial Revolution, people produced goods by hand. Afterward, the availability of machines as well as improvements in water power, increased use of steam power, and the switch from wood and other biofuels to coal caused mechanised manufacturing to boom. The Industrial Revolution also affected the agricultural industry (see **Agricultural Revolution**) with the invention of farming machines that made it possible to farm larger areas. It also freed up workers to work in other areas of the economy.

Industrialised Seed Oils – See **Seed Oils**

Inflammation – A part of the body's system of defence against **pathogens** and the body's response to an infection. The classic symptoms of inflammation are redness, swelling, heat, pain, and loss of function.

There are two kinds of inflammation: acute and chronic. Acute inflammation is generally a short-term response to a harmful stimulus that recedes once the **anti-inflammatory** process neutralises the threat; chronic inflammation is a prolonged inflammation that can lead to destruction of healthy tissue and a variety of diseases, including anything with an '*itis*' suffix, such as arthritis, periodontitis, and meningitis. Inflammation is also linked to **allergies**, asthma, cardiovascular disease, and **autoimmune diseases**. There is evidence linking autoimmune disease to chronic inflammation of the gut.

The **Paleo diet**, and, in particular, the **autoimmune protocol**, can help to rebalance the **gut flora** and reduce inflammation, thus alleviating or even eliminating inflammation and the problems caused by it. See **Systemic Inflammation**

Insulin – A hormone produced by the pancreas that lowers the amount of glucose in the blood. Fat cells are not used for energy when there is insulin present. See *Glucagon*

Insulin Resistance – A state where elevated *insulin* and abnormally low *insulin sensitivity* over a prolonged period leads to an inability for the body to regulate normal *blood glucose levels* as the body's cells fail to react to insulin. Insulin resistance can lead to *type II diabetes* and is associated with a host of conditions such as *metabolic syndrome, obesity, high blood pressure,* heart disease, *osteoporosis,* and *cancer.*

Insulin Sensitivity – Describes how sensitive the body is to the effects of *insulin.* If sensitivity is low, the body will compensate by producing more insulin. Many people live with high levels of circulating insulin because of the high levels of refined and processed carbohydrates in the modern diet. Insulin sensitivity can be increased through physical activity. See *Insulin Resistance*

Intermittent Fasting (IF) – The term that describes alternating periods of little or no food consumption (*fasting*) with regular food consumption. The fasting periods may be several days long for some methods and several hours for others.

Ancient hunter-gatherers often ate intermittently due to the availability of food. The human body evolved on a cycle of eating and fasting, with the routine of consuming three meals (plus snacks and grazing) daily being a relatively recent eating pattern. Studies suggest intermittent fasting helps the body to rejuvenate and repair, promotes the burning of fat stores as fuel and thereby promotes overall health. Evidence of a range of therapeutic benefits include:

- Reduction in *inflammation*
- Improvements in circulating *blood sugar* and blood lipid levels
- Reduction of blood pressure
- Improvements in body composition
- Improvements in *insulin sensitivity*
- Protection against cardiovascular disease
- Reduction in levels of *visceral fat*

Some animal studies show that mice who fast intermittently consume fewer calories overall than those who eat freely. Research also demonstrates that rodents and insects who fast may live longer, healthier lives than those who do not.

Some popular methods include fasting for twenty-four hours and then eating normally for twenty-four hours, fasting no more than two days a week. Other methods suggest fasting 14 to 16 hours a day and then eating during the other eight to ten hours, known as a *compressed eating* or *time-restricted* window. The *5:2 diet* uses a form of fasting where you eat normally for five days and then restrict calories for two days, with a goal of 500 calories a day for women and 600 for men. More extreme versions of IF may include fasting periods as long as thirty-six hours.

Intestinal Permeability – See *Leaky Gut Syndrome*

Intolerance – See *Food Intolerance*

Inuit – The Inuit are a group of aboriginal people who live in the Arctic regions of the United States, Canada, and Greenland. The Inuit fish and hunt their food and consume a diet that is as much as 75 per cent fat during the winter months and have very low incidence of cardiovascular disease.

Iodine – A mineral found mainly in foods from the ocean. Most of the world's iodine is found in the oceans, so good food sources are fish, *shellfish*, seaweed, cod, and scallops. Countries such as the United States, Switzerland, and Denmark add iodine to salt products to ensure adequate iodine intake. The United Kingdom does not. If you are *deficient*, a supplement of 100 to 150 mcg of potassium iodide can help.

Iodine Deficiency – The *World Health Organization* says that *iodine* deficiency is the biggest cause of mental impairment. It has been linked to low IQ, fatigue, miscarriage, and problems with the thyroid. Serious cases can lead to *hypothyroidism*.

Iron – A mineral that is essential to all life. Iron is a major component of *haemoglobin* and also forms a core part of proteins involved in *metabolism*, immune response, and the production of *neurotransmitters*. Too much iron in the blood can lead to constipation, and improper iron storage is a factor in diseases such as Alzheimer's and

Parkinson's. Low blood iron can lead to anaemia. *Organ meats* and *leafy greens* are especially rich sources of iron.

Some foods can change the amount of iron that is absorbed from a meal. Eating cooked meat with iron-rich *vegetables*, for example, will increase the amount of iron absorbed from the vegetables. Other foods that increase iron absorption include oranges, kiwis, carrots, tomatoes, red grapes, and peaches.

Antinutrients, especially *tannins*, can negatively affect iron absorption. Blueberries, spinach, eggs, milk, *walnuts*, coffee, chocolate, tea, wheat bran, strawberries, and herbs all decrease iron absorption. One egg can reduce the iron absorbed from a meal by 28 per cent. In the United Kingdom, 46 per cent of girls aged eleven to eighteen do not get enough iron. See *Antinutrients*

Iron Overload – A detrimental accumulation of iron in the body. A review of over 2,000 scientific papers by Douglas Kell at the University of Manchester examining iron and disease concluded that iron overload contributes significantly to a host of today's *chronic diseases*.

J

"SO MANY PEOPLE SPEND THEIR HEALTH GAINING WEALTH, AND THEN HAVE TO SPEND THEIR WEALTH TO REGAIN THEIR HEALTH."

—A.J. REB MATERI

JERF – An acronym meaning *'Just Eat Real Food'*. This powerful and common sense term was coined by Sean Croxton from a podcast called the Underground Wellness Show.

Jetlag – Jetlag occurs when the ***circadian rhythm*** or body clock is disrupted by crossing a number of time zones. The symptoms can include fatigue, disorientation and an inability to ***sleep***. Methods to reduce the effects of jetlag include the following:

- Before you travel, adjust your wake and sleep cycle to be as close as possible to your destination's time zone. So if you are travelling west, wake up one hour later and go to bed one hour later than usual for three consecutive days. For example, if you usually wake at 7 o'clock and go to bed at 10 o'clock, then three days before travel, wake up at 8 o'clock and go to sleep by 11 o'clock. The next day it would be 9 o'clock and 12 o'clock, and so on. If travelling east, do the reverse.

- On the day of your flight, fast immediately before and during the flight, drink plenty of water during the flight, and avoiding ***caffeinated*** and ***alcoholic*** beverages.

- On arrival, eat as soon as possible and ***exercise*** during daylight hours, preferably outdoors, where you can get natural sunlight, too.
- Stick to the local time in terms of eating, activity, and sleeping as best you can. If you need a nap during the day, sleep no more than twenty minutes to avoid affecting sleep later at night.

Juicing (juice) – A popular way of getting more ***vegetables*** and ***fruits*** into the daily diet. Proponents of juicing claim that the juicing process makes the nutrients easier for the body to absorb. However, juicing also results in a drink that includes very little of the fibrous parts of the whole fruit or vegetable, meaning it has an increased amount of ***sugar*** and thus a high ***glycaemic index***.

See ***Smoothies***

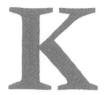

"I WANT TO TALK TO YOU ABOUT ONE OF THE BIGGEST MYTHS IN MEDICINE, AND THAT IS THE IDEA THAT ALL WE NEED ARE MORE MEDICAL BREAKTHROUGHS AND THEN ALL OF OUR PROBLEMS WILL BE SOLVED."

—QUYEN NGUYEN

Kefir – A *fermented* milk drink that boasts a wide variety of *probiotic* bacteria. It also contains beneficial yeasts such as saccharomyces kefir and torula kefir. These two yeasts are said to be able to fight against undesirable *yeast* overgrowths in the gut, such as *candida albicans*.

Ketoacidosis – A potentially fatal condition that can occur in type I diabetics because they don't produce insulin. Not to be confused with nutritional *ketosis* that occurs when the body uses fat for fuel. See *Ketogenic Diet*

Ketogenesis – The process used by the body to manufacture *ketones*, which allow the body to use stored fat as energy. Ketogenesis occurs in the *mitochondria* of liver cells, and the resultant ketones allow the body to pull energy from lipids or fats. See *Ketogenic Diet*

Ketogenic Diet – A specialised diet traditionally used to treat epilepsy in children, as ketones have been found to have a calming effect on the brain. The ratios of fat to protein to carbohydrate are different from traditional diets. People on a ketogenic diet consume four times as much fat as protein and carbohydrates combined. It restricts carb intake to between 25 and 60 grams a day. Eating this way puts the body into *ketosis*, which enables it to convert stored fat into energy.

Randomised trials demonstrate that children who follow this diet may experience up to a 50 per cent reduction in the number of seizures they have. There are trials underway such as the Recharge (REduced CarboHydrAtes for Resistant Growth Tumours) trial by Dr Eugene Fine, which looks at the benefits of the ketogenic diet in inhibiting cancer growth. There are also randomised trials where ketosis is used to manage health conditions such as type II diabetes and metabolic syndrome. See *Ketones, Ketogenesis, LCHF*

Ketones – Produced when the body burns fat for fuel. *Mitochondria* in the liver produce ketones during a process called *ketogenesis*. Ketones move from the liver into the bloodstream and enable the body to use stored fat as an alternative energy source. The ketone pathway was developed as a way to provide humans with energy in times of famine.

Ketosis – A metabolic state that occurs either during a fast or a prolonged *low-carbohydrate* diet. Sometimes referred to as the body's fat-burning state, ketosis happens when the body has used the glycogen stored in the liver, which triggers the release of *ketones* into the bloodstream; the body then uses the ketones for energy. The body now uses stored fat for energy, which can lead to fat loss. See *Ketogenic Diet*

Kidney – See *Organ Meats*

Kimchi (Kimchee) – A traditional *fermented* Korean food made of *vegetables* (usually white cabbage) with a variety of seasonings.

Kitavans – A group of people native to the island of Kitava in Papua New Guinea. Because of their remote locations, the Kitavans eat a diet free of *processed foods* and is a cross between a *hunter-gatherer* diet and an early agricultural diet. The bulk of their diet consists of *tubers* such as *yams* and cassava, *fruits*, *vegetables*, fish, and *coconut.*

See *Staffan Lindeberg*

Kombucha – A drink made by fermenting sweetened tea with a live culture. The culture feeds off the tea and sugar to create Kombucha. It is slightly effervescent, so it makes a great alternative to carbonated soft drinks. The *fermentation* process leaves behind *probiotics*, active enzymes, and *antioxidants*.

Konner, Mel – See *History of the Paleo Diet*

L

"PIONEERING SPIRIT SHOULD CONTINUE, NOT
TO CONQUER THE PLANET OR SPACE, BUT
RATHER TO IMPROVE THE QUALITY OF LIFE."

—BERTRAND PICCARD

Lactase – An enzyme that breaks down the sugar *lactose* found in *dairy* products. Typically humans produce less lactase after weaning, which can lead to *lactose intolerance*.

Lactose – A carbohydrate found in most *dairy* products. See *Lactose Intolerance*

Lactose Intolerance – The inability of the body to break down lactose. Typically, dairy intolerance is related to a lack of the enzyme *lactase*. Lactose intolerance ranges from five per cent in Northern Europeans to more than ninety per cent in those of African and Asian descent. Milk protein *intolerance* is another common dairy intolerance and occurs when an individual has problems breaking down milk proteins such as *casein* and *whey*. See *Food Intolerance*

Lard – Cooking fat made from rendered pig fat. Lard has a mild pork smell and roughly even levels of saturated fats (40 per cent) and monounsaturated fats (45 per cent).

Lard is solid at room temperature, very heat-resistant, and a good choice for cooking, especially frying. Obtain lard from pastured sources. See *Tallow*

Laughter – Laughter is medicine. Studies have found that people who laugh more readily and frequently could improve artery function, have a lower risk of heart disease and a lower risk of suffering heart attacks. According to research at the University of Athens (Greece) laughter reduces the stiffness of the arteries, a cardiovascular disease risk indicator. They also found it resulted in lower levels of the stress hormone *cortisol*. Other research suggests that laughter causes the blood vessels to dilate (*expand*), which improves blood flow and reduces blood pressure. Benefits of laughter include:

- Boosts levels of endorphins (our bodies' natural painkillers) which increases pain tolerance
- Reduces pro-inflammatory cytokines and increases anti-inflammatory cytokines (*inflammation*)
- Reduces skin reactions to allergens during tests and lowers levels of antibodies
- Improves *sleep quality*
- Reduces blood glucose levels
- Increases levels of HDL cholesterol

LCHF – Stands for 'Low-Carb High-Fat' where the proportion of fat is around 80 per cent of the diet and the maximum threshold for carbohydrate intake is 50 to 150 grams of carbs per day – depending on lifestyle and activity levels. See *Ketogenic Diet*

LDL (Low-Density Lipoprotein) – See *Cholesterol, Blood Work*

Lead – One of three heavy metal contaminants, along with *cadmium* and *mercury*, for which the European Commission has set maximum permitted contamination levels in food. Lead is banned in the European Union, and the regulation of its use in pipes and paints has led to reduced lead exposure. However, all the lead released over the years has made it into the soil, so we end up eating it in our food. The main culprits are cereals, with vegetables and tap water also contributing to the ingestion of lead.

In 2010, the European Food Safety Authority concluded that there is no safe blood lead level. Even at low levels, lead is associated with lower IQ and anaemia, with children most at risk.

Leafy Greens – Dark green leafy *vegetables* including kale, spring greens (collard greens), mustard greens, dandelion greens, spinach, turnip greens, callaloo, and rocket (arugula). They are good sources of minerals such as *iron* and *calcium*, and good sources of *vitamins* such as *vitamin A, C,* and *K.*

Leaky Gut Syndrome (Leaky Gut) – A term for gastrointestinal issues caused when the small intestinal walls become permeable, allowing substances to leak from the digestive tract into the bloodstream. These holes allow partially digested proteins to enter the bloodstream, possibly triggering the body to attack its own cells because it recognizes them as *pathogens* through the process of *molecular mimicry.* If this process continues, it can create even more *inflammation* and increase the likelihood of more small intestinal permeability and *autoimmune disease.*

Some of the major causes of leaky gut include *alcohol, NSAIDs, gluten, dairy, legumes,* and *nightshades,* chronic *stress,* and gut *dysbiosis.* The process of healing will involve establishing and removing what's contributing to systemic inflammation and intestinal permeability. Whether it's a particular food or a multitude of factors and then undergoing a process of elimination.

Lectins – Proteins found in plants such as *grains*, *seeds*, and *legumes*, as well as those in the *nightshade* family (such as the tomato and potato); they protect the plant's seeds. Lectins can get stuck to the intestine and are detected as foreign invaders by the *immune system*. This can lead to *leaky gut*, autoimmune issues, and *insulin resistance.* Research has shown that lectins found in most plants are harmless, but some lectins found in the list above are harmful to humans. See *Antinutrients*

Legumes – A plant, fruit or seeds of the Fabaceae family. Many *vegetarians* use legumes as a substitute for the protein found in meat. They are not a part of the *Paleo diet* because they contain *antinutrients* such as *lectins* and phytates, both of which may hinder the body's ability to absorb nutrients. In addition, legumes may cause digestive issues (see FODMAP), thereby contributing to *leaky gut syndrome*, *irritable bowel* *syndrome*, and other digestive disorders. Some examples of legumes are fresh and dried peas, peanuts, alfalfa, lentils, kidney beans, liquorice, carob, and soya beans.

Leptin – A hormone produced by fat cells in the body. Leptin helps to regulate appetite and burn fat, telling you when you have had enough food. It is also called '*the satiety hormone*'. See **Leptin Resistance**, **Ghrelin**, **Sleep**

Leptin Resistance – Occurs when the body becomes resistant to *leptin*. This can occur when there is too much leptin in the blood, which may contribute to weight gain and *obesity*, as the body cannot tell when it is full. By helping to maintain a hormone balance, improving body composition to healthier body fat levels, and focussing on improving *sleep* quality the *Paleo lifestyle* may help to recalibrate the body's reactions to leptin.

Lifestyle – The way in which a person lives and a key determinant of one's health. Identical twin studies (i.e. twins who have the same heredity and identical genes) have found that genetic factors explain around a 25 per cent variation in lifespan, meaning that 75 per cent of gene expression and the impact on health are based on environmental factors and lifestyle decisions. See *Paleo Lifestyle*

Lifestyle Diseases – (noncommunicable diseases) are illnesses whose frequency and severity have increased as the world becomes more industrialised. Examples of lifestyle diseases include cardiovascular disease, Alzheimer's, arthritis, *diabetes*, *depression*, and certain cancers. Lifestyle diseases have been identified by the *World Health Organisation* in the *Global Status Report on Noncommunicable Diseases 2014* as the leading cause of death and disability globally, responsible for 68 per cent of the world's deaths in 2012.

See *Chronic Disease*

Lindeberg, Staffan – A Swedish physician best known for writing *The Kitava Study*, a study of the eating habits of the native people of Kitava. His research is relevant to the *Paleo diet*, as studying the eating habits of existing *hunter-gatherer* societies may help us to better understand how our early ancestors ate.

See *History of the Paleo Diet*

Lipid Hypothesis – A theory that says that lowering the amount of lipids in plasma will reduce the chances of developing heart disease. While the idea of lowering lipids has been around since the early 1900s, this theory gained popularity in 1976 when a group of twenty-one scientists participated in a survey about the link between *cholesterol* levels and cardiovascular disease. See *History of Fat*

Lipids – Any one of several different kinds of naturally occurring molecules. While most people associate the word '*lipid*' with fat, fat is only one type of lipid. Others include wax, triglycerides, and vitamins *A*, *D*, *E*, and *K*, which are *fat soluble*.

Liver – See *Organ Meats*

Low-Carb – See *Low-Carb Diet*

Low-Carb Diet (Low Carbohydrate Diet) – Also known as '*Low-Carb*', the Low-Carb diet is a way of eating that restricts carbohydrates to less than 20 per cent of total *macronutrient* intake.

Low-Fat Diet – A diet that reduces overall fat intake. Low-fat diets have been popular for years, but there are some disadvantages to following such a diet. Many foods that have reduced fat also include additional sugars, salt, and preservatives to make them taste better. Also, the body needs a certain amount of *fat* in order to be healthy.

Low-FODMAP Diet – A diet limiting *FODMAP* consumption to help alleviate or eliminate symptoms of Irritable Bowel Syndrome (*IBS*).

Low-Histamine Diet – A diet limiting *histamine* exposure from foods to help reduce or eliminate symptoms of histamine intolerance. Foods to avoid include *nuts*, *chocolate*, *alcohol*, *vinegar*, and *shellfish*.

Lunch – Paleo lunches do not need to be complicated. One simple way to make healthy lunches for the week is to make a big salad of mixed *vegetables*. Each day, simply add a serving of Paleo *protein* (wild-caught *fish*, *pastured beef*, etc.), dress the salad with *olive oil*

Lupus – An *autoimmune disease* that can affect the skin, joints, kidneys, brain and other organs.

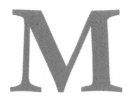

"THE SUPERIOR DOCTOR PREVENTS SICKNESS;
THE MEDIOCRE DOCTOR ATTENDS TO
IMPENDING SICKNESS;
THE INFERIOR DOCTOR TREATS ACTUAL
SICKNESS."

—CHINESE PROVERB

Macronutrients – One of two distinct groups of nutrients (the other being *micronutrients*) that provides the energy and building blocks we need to construct and maintain every cell and organ in the body. Macronutrients (macro = big) are nutrients that the human body requires in large amounts—on the order of grams—in order to thrive, namely *protein*, *fat*, *carbohydrates*, and fibre. The following is a breakdown of our *hunter-gatherer* ancestors' macronutrients:

- Protein: 25 to 35 per cent
- Carbohydrates: 25 to 40 per cent
- Fat: 30 to 45 per cent

Magnesium – The second-most abundant *micronutrient* inside human cells. Sufficient magnesium is vital to human health, as it serves hundreds of functions in the body. It is an essential *mineral* that must be supplied through diet, although it can be obtained by *supplementation* or topical applications (where it is absorbed through the skin). In the United States, teenagers and the elderly often get too little magnesium, partly due to a diet high in processed food for the former and poor absorption of the mineral for the latter. Magnesium deficiency is linked to asthma, anxiety, *osteoporosis*, and *diabetes*.

Foods that are high in magnesium include dark leafy greens, mackerel, *seeds*, nuts such as *Brazil nuts*, and avocados. If you take a magnesium supplement, take it in a chelated form such as magnesium citrate, which is easier for the body to absorb. Too much magnesium in supplement form can have a laxative effect.

Magnesium's role in muscle function acts as a muscle relaxant and can lessen the discomfort caused by *muscle soreness* (DOMS) after exercise (for example bathing in Epsom salts) or pain caused by womb contractions during a period. A study showed that taking 360mg of magnesium for three days, beginning the day before a period starts, helped reduce cramps. Other trials report magnesium as more effective than a placebo when it comes to period pain relief.

MCT Oil (Medium-Chain Triglycerides) – MCTs are medium-chain fatty acids found in *coconut* and palm oils. Consumption of MCT oil may help with *weight loss* and calorie burning. See *Coconut Oil*

ME (Myalgic Encephalopathy) – See *Chronic Fatigue Syndrome*

Meal Frequency – Consume two to three hearty meals a day and avoid snacking.

Meat Consumption – In 2013, the EPIC (European Prospective Investigation into Cancer and Nutrition) trial, a large-scale research involving more than half a million people for nearly fifteen years, found little or no connection between *meat* consumption and cancer or heart disease. It factored for *smoking*, *fitness*, *BMI*, and education levels. The study found no association between red meat and ill health; however, processed meat was considered to be an issue. The study found that for every 50 grams of *processed* meat consumed daily, the risk of early death from all causes increased by 18 per cent.

Meats – Choose organic, *grass-fed*, *free-range* meat. These grass-fed variants are more expensive but have a healthier nutrient profile and no *antibiotics*, hormones, or fillers. Good sources of meat include beef, buffalo, lamb, goat, mutton, turkey, and chicken. See *Game*

Mediterranean Diet – A popular diet based on the traditional foods eaten by people living around the Mediterranean Sea. The Mediterranean diet is based on eating *fruits* and *vegetables*, whole *grains*, *fish*, and healthy *fats* like olive oil.

There are studies that suggest the *Paleo diet* has a greater positive impact on health than the Mediterranean diet. One such study conducted by *Dr. Staffan Lindeberg* in 2009 over a 6-month period using a *crossover design* (with half of the subjects following one diet for a 3-month period and then switching to the other diet for 3-months). The Paleo diet had improved results in relation to *weight loss*, *waist circumference*, *blood pressure*, *triglycerides*, *blood glucose* and *hbA1c* in comparison with the Mediterranean diet.

Melatonin – A *hormone* that helps regulate *sleep cycles* and *circadian rhythms*. Melatonin is also an *antioxidant* and part of the body's immune response system. A deficiency of melatonin may lead to trouble sleeping. While melatonin is available as a dietary supplement, the effects of taking it long term are still in question. See *Sleep*, *Sleep Tips*

Mercury – One of three heavy metal contaminants, along with *cadmium* and *lead*, for which the European Commission has set maximum permitted contamination levels in food. Mercury accumulates in the food chain, and top-predator fish (such as tuna and salmon) are our main dietary sources. Too much mercury can lead to developmental damage in babies and small children. Mercury intake can be reduced by limiting top-predator fish and eating smaller fish such as sardines, anchovies, and so on. See *Vaccinations*

Meta-Analysis – A classification of *research* where statistical techniques are used to combine the findings from two or more independent studies. Meta-analyses aim to encompass all relevant studies and to find robust consensus amongst the body of evidence to determine the relative effect of treatment. However, meta-analyses are only as good as the quality of the underlying studies included in the analysis. See *Systematic Review*

Metabolic Syndrome – A group of factors that contribute to an increased chance of cardiovascular disease. The factors are abdominal obesity, elevated *triglycerides*, low HDL *cholesterol*, *high blood pressure*, and high fasting *blood sugar* levels. See *Insulin Resistance*

Metabolism – The process that powers body and mind by converting what we eat into fuel. It involves a complex system of hormones, enzymes, and processes that govern how efficiently we burn that fuel. See *BMR*

Micro-organism (microorganism) – An organism that is so small that it is invisible to the naked eye. There are three types of micro-organism viruses, bacteria and fungi. Some micro-organisms are harmful to humans (*pathogens*), but others are beneficial such as *L. plantarum* found in many *fermented food* products and *probiotics*. See *dysbiosis*

Microbe – See *Micro-organism*

Microbiome – A term coined by Joshua Lederberg to describe the *micro-organisms* that inhabit our bodies.

While the entire microbiome in a human body weighs about seven ounces, it contains ten times as many microbes as there are human cells in the body. The balance of microbes in the microbiome is crucial to human health. An unhealthy mix of microbes may be a contributing factor to obesity as well as to *autoimmune diseases* such as fibromyalgia, *rheumatoid arthritis*, *diabetes*, and even cancer.

See *probiotics, fermented foods, dysbiosis*

Micronutrients – One of two distinct groups of nutrients (the other being *macronutrients*) that provide the energy and building blocks we need to construct and maintain every cell and organ in the body. *Vitamins* and *minerals* are examples of micronutrients (micro = small) that the body needs to perform a wide range of functions, such as essential chemical reactions, that make it possible for the body to move. Examples include *vitamin C, iron*, chromium, copper, *iodine*, manganese, *selenium*, and *zinc*.

The human body requires far fewer micronutrients than macronutrients, on the order of milligrams (thousandths of a gram) or micrograms (millionths of a gram). Getting sufficient micronutrients decreases maternal, and infant mortality and increases average IQ and work capacity.

Microorganism – See *Micro-organism*

Minimalist Shoes (Barefoot Shoes) – *Conventional wisdom* informs us that shoes (especially training shoes) should provide extra support and stability to reduce injury. However, there is limited evidence that regular shoes are a major cause of many foot ailments such as flatfoot and collapsed arches. They also change our natural gait and balance when standing, walking and running, causing many of the foot, hip, knee, and back problems that plague us today. Minimalist shoes are designed to combat these issues by allowing for a more natural gait with minimal support. These shoes often include zero-drop heals, anatomical width (including a wide toe box to allow for natural splaying of the toes with increased balance), and increased flexibility in the sole. Minimalist shoes provide a sensation closer to being barefoot without going barefoot. See *Barefoot Running*

Mindfulness – An approach in which the practitioner focuses full attention on the present moment. Mindfulness reduces stress and anxiety and improves well-being.

Minerals – Minerals are important for health. Your body uses minerals for different functions, including building bones, manufacturing hormones and heartbeat regulation. The six essential minerals include calcium, magnesium, sodium, potassium, chloride and phosphorus; trace minerals include copper, chromium, fluoride, iodine, iron, manganese, *selenium*, and zinc. See *Micronutrients*

Mint – A *herb* rich in *vitamin C* and also contains *magnesium*, *iron*, *potassium*, and *calcium*. Aids in digestion and promotes oral health.

Mitochondria – Tiny compartments in cells that keep the cells full of energy. Mitochondria are called the *'powerhouse'* of cells.

Molecular Mimicry – A theory that proteins manufactured in the body may sometimes mimic the protein structure of foreign objects such as proteins in food. See *Leaky Gut*

Monosodium Glutamate – See *MSG*

Monounsaturated Fats – Fats that are found in foods such as olives and avocados. Research shows that these oils may improve *insulin sensitivity* and help to regulate *blood sugar.*

Monsanto – A large international agricultural company headquartered in St. Louis, Missouri. (U.S.) Monsanto is a leading producer of genetically modified seeds or *GMOs*, and also manufacture a popular pesticide called Roundup. Monsanto typifies the *Big Agra* mentality. They have a large market share, and that makes it difficult and more expensive for small farmers to purchase seeds elsewhere.

Monsanto's approach to food production is in direct contrast with the *Paleo diet.* Monsanto seeks to modify and homogenise nature. Altering crops and using pesticides may both contribute to illnesses, including cancer. Monsanto's virtual monopoly of corn has had a negative impact on honey production in Mexico because the biodiversity of the area has suffered and so have the bees. The Paleo diet emphasizes natural, unmodified foods, which are healthier for humans, animals, and the planet.

Mood – A particular state of mind or emotion that can be influenced by several factors, including *blood sugar levels* and the level of neurotransmitters such as serotonin and dopamine. See *Depression, Laughter*

Moore, Jimmy – An author and advocate of a low-carb, high-fat diet *ketogenic* diet. Runs a popular weekly podcast with experts in diet, fitness and health, called *Livin' La Vida Low Carb.*

Motor Cortex – The principal part of the brain that controls *movement.* The role of the motor cortex is to generate neural impulses to execute motor function, from talking to *walking.*

Movement – A recognition that in the broadest sense that physical activity in the widest variety of natural forms is vital and healthful, through a range of locomotion, regular change of position and a combination of postures. See *Sedentary Behaviour*

MSG (Monosodium Glutamate E621) – A chemical additive that enhances the taste of food. MSG is considered to be a *neurotoxin* as large doses are believed to cause headaches and other issues. There is controversy surrounding MSG intolerance because there is a naturally occurring form of MSG (*glutamate*) that acts as a *neurotransmitter* safely within the body. MSG is often added to processed and fast foods to stimulate a craving for that particular food.

Multiple Sclerosis (MS) – An *autoimmune disease* that affects the brain and spinal cord, caused by damage to the myelin sheath. The nerve damage is caused by chronic *inflammation* where the body's own immune cells attack the nervous system.
See *Terry Wahls*

Muscle Soreness (after *Exercise*) – See *DOMS*

Mushrooms – The spore-bearing body of a fungus, typically found growing from the earth or directly from its food source. Mushrooms are an excellent source of *B vitamins*, copper, *selenium*, and other essential *minerals*.

Mycotoxin – The *toxins* produced by moulds, which are members of the fungi family. Foods stored in heat and humidity are a breeding ground for mycotoxins, which can cause a variety of health problems such as damage to the nervous system. They may also be *carcinogenic*. There are several different kinds of mycotoxins, including *aflatoxins*.

N

"A MAN'S HEALTH CAN BE JUDGED BY WHICH
HE TAKES TWO AT A TIME - PILLS OR STAIRS."

—JOAN WELSH

N=1 – A term that refers to self-experimentation, where N stands for the size of the sample. It is also used as an abbreviation for 'in my experience'. The concept of self-experimentation is not a new one. It can be an important part of scientific discovery, as it provides first-hand experience of the effects of an experiment. See *Biohacking*

Nap – A brief period of *sleep*, usually taken during daytime. To optimise napping and to reduce the impact on bedtime sleep late, aim for either twenty minutes (this avoids entering a deep *sleep cycle*) or ninety minutes (this is roughly the time needed to complete one iteration of a full sleep cycle).

Naturally Raised – A term coined by the *USDA*. '*Naturally raised*' is a voluntary standard for farm animals that have been raised with no *growth hormones* or antibiotics and has not been fed animal by-products. The meat is also minimally processed in comparison to intense farming practices. See *Factory Farmed, Organic*

Naturally Reared – A term used in the United Kingdom to denote that traditional farming practices are followed, including natural weaning, *pastured* on grass, living outdoors all year round, without the use of any chemicals or antibiotics. See *Factory Farmed, Organic*

Neolithic (New Stone Age) – A period of human history beginning in approximately 10,000 BC and ending between 4,500 and 2,000 BC. The Neolithic Period is the last part of the Stone Age and marks the human transition to the *Agricultural Revolution.*

Neolithic Revolution – See *Agricultural Revolution*

Neurotoxins, neurotoxic – A natural or artificial substance that can cause damage to the nervous system. High levels or prolonged exposure to neurotoxins can lead to neurotoxicity which can result in the death of neurons (nerve cells) in the brain and other parts of the nervous system, leading to symptoms including headaches, cognitive issues, and numbness of limbs. See *Toxins*

Neurotransmitters – Chemicals that send a signal from one brain cell (*neuron*) to another. Some examples of neurotransmitters include amino acids such as glutamate and aspartate, monoamines such as *dopamine* and *serotonin*, and peptides such as somatostatin.

Niacin – See *Vitamin B3*

Nicotine – An *alkaloid* stimulant found in the *nightshade* family of plants and a mood-altering drug that can act as both a stimulant and a relaxant which is likely to be a major contributing factor to the addictive-forming properties of tobacco and *smoking*. Nicotine is addictive. Nicotine also increases blood pressure and heart rate.

Nightshades (*Solanaceae*) – A family of flowering plants many of which are edible. Examples of nightshades are *potatoes*, tomatoes, aubergine (eggplant), sweet (bell/capsicum), chilli and habanero peppers, tomatillos, and gooseberries. Some members of the family contain toxic *alkaloids*, for example, *tobacco* is also a member of the nightshade family, as is the highly poisonous plant belladonna (deadly nightshade). The *autoimmune* *protocol* version of the Paleo diet does not include nightshades because there is evidence showing they may contribute to *inflammation* and thus worsen symptoms for *autoimmune diseases* such as *rheumatoid arthritis*. See *Nicotine*

Nitrates – Compounds made of nitrogen and oxygen. Many fertilizers contain nitrates because they are biodegradable. Nitrates are also used as preservatives in cured meats such as bacon. They are present in root vegetables and leafy vegetables and are not usually harmful unless they are consumed in excessive quantities. Some health risks associated with nitrate toxicity include migraines, blue baby syndrome, cancer, and leukaemia. See *Nitrites*

Nitrites – Compounds that are very similar, but not identical, to *nitrates* and are not commonly found in nature. The food industry uses nitrites as a preservative for cured meats, such as sausages and hot dogs because they help to prevent the growth of bacteria and give the meat a pink colour. The use of nitrites is controversial because, during *cooking*, they may react with amino acids to form a ***carcinogenic*** substance called nitrosamine. Nearly all nitrites consumed come from cured meats. See ***Nitrates***

Non-Coeliac Gluten Sensitivity (U.S. Non-Celiac Gluten Sensitivity) – A term used to describe individuals who experience symptoms similar to those with coeliac disease such as headache, joint pain, and *'brain fog'* yet who lack the same antibodies and intestinal damage experienced with an autoimmune response. In other words, individuals with non-coeliac gluten sensitivity would not test positive for coeliac disease based on blood tests. The onset of symptoms is hours to days after gluten exposure. Symptoms disappear with a ***gluten-free*** diet. See ***Coeliac Disease***, ***Gluten***

Noncommunicable Diseases – See ***Lifestyle Diseases***

Nose to Tail – A term used to describe consuming every part of an animal, including those parts not conventionally included in the human diet. These parts include ***organ meats*** such as hearts, kidneys, and livers as well as tongue, ears, and trotters (hooves). The ***Paleo***

diet incorporates these animal parts, which are often very nutrient dense.

Nourishing Traditions – A cookbook by Sally Fallon and Susan Enig, first published in 1999. *Nourishing Traditions* explores the importance of animal fat to the human diet and the dangers of *processed foods* and includes many recipes. See *Weston A. Price*

NSAID (Non-Steroidal Anti-Inflammatory Drug) – Drugs typically used for pain relief and to reduce swelling and inflammation. Examples of NSAIDs include aspirin, ibuprofen and diclofenac. See *Leaky Gut Syndrome*

Nut Butters – Butter substitutes made by crushing nuts, nut butters include *almond* butter, *cashew* butter, hazelnut butter, *walnut* butter, and macadamia butter. Make sure to read the labels to be sure the products don't contain added sugar or *trans fats*. See *Nuts*

Nut Flours – Flour substitutes made by grinding up the so-called '*cake*' that is left after pressing oil from *nuts*. *Gluten-free* recipes sometimes include nut flours as a substitute for wheat flour, both in baking and for breading meats and *vegetables*. Nut flours contain high amounts of *polyunsaturated fats* such as *omega-6*, and *phytates*, which reduce the absorption of *minerals*. Nuts may also contribute to *inflammation*, and it is best to consume them in moderation. See *Nuts*

Nutrient Density (Quality of Food) – A measure of the amount of nutrients in a food relative to the amount of energy it produces. Food that is high in nutrients and low in calories is nutrient dense.

Nutrient Interaction – The way nutrients work together. A nutrient does not work in isolation, and a nutrient has multiple functions. For example, if you consume an iron-rich food such as steak together with a sweet (bell) pepper, the vitamin C in the sweet pepper can better absorb the iron. However, if you also eat berries at the same mealtime, they contain tannins which can impede iron absorption. An excess of one nutrient (or the consumption of *antinutrients*) can interfere with the absorption of another. As long as you eat a varied diet of nutrient-rich, whole foods and have a healthy gut, you should get all the nutrients your body needs.

Nutrition – The science of how the body takes in and uses food and *water*. Nutrition is the study of the dietary requirements of people as they relate to health, disease and wellbeing.

Nuts – Nuts are the fruits of the parent plant, in most cases. Examples of nuts include *almonds*, *Brazil nuts*, chestnuts, hazelnuts, macadamias, *walnuts*, *cashews*, pecans, and pistachios. Despite their name, *peanuts* are a *legume*, not a nut. Nuts are an excellent source of *monounsaturated fats* (MUFAs). Diets rich in *polyunsaturated fatty acids* (PUFAs) are associated with improved fat *metabolism* and a lesser incidence of cardiovascular disease; however most of the PUFAs in nuts are *omega-6*. We should be mindful of maintaining our *omega-3:6 ratio*. Since nuts are extremely calorie dense, consuming them in moderation is the key if you are focusing on *weight loss*. People following the *autoimmune protocol* should not eat nuts.

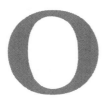

"THE PART CAN NEVER BE WELL UNLESS THE
WHOLE IS WELL."

—PLATO

Obesity – A medical term for being severely overweight to the point that the excess weight has an adverse effect on overall health. Obesity is defined as being 40 per cent above his or her ideal weight. In most Western countries, obesity means having a **BMI** (body mass index) of over 30. Obesity increases the risk of developing many **lifestyle diseases** and related health problems. Research shows that it can be beneficial to lose even 10 per cent of your body weight if you are overweight or obese. Losing weight can decrease **blood pressure** and **blood sugar** and take pressure off overstressed joints.

The worldwide obesity epidemic is a relatively new phenomenon. The Organization for Economic Cooperation and Development (OECD), in the report *Obesity and the Economics of Prevention: Fit Not Fat*, stated that in 1980 obesity rates were well below 10%. Since then, the rates have doubled or tripled in the world's 33 richest countries. In 2008, 1.5 billion adults over 20 years old were overweight, globally. Of these, over 200 million men and nearly 300 million women were obese. In comparison, there are 870 million people who are chronically hungry. A recent report by Trust for America's Health and the Robert Wood Johnson Foundation forecasts that more than half of Americans will be obese by 2030. See *Overweight*

Oestrogen (U.S. Estrogen) – A group of hormones which mainly promote the development and maintenance of female characteristics in the body. Oestrogens are the primary sex hormone in women, but men naturally produce small quantities of oestrogen too. Saturated fat contains *cholesterol*, which the body converts to sex *hormones* including oestrogens.

Women with ultra-low body fat such as athletes or those driven to be ultra-lean often do not produce sufficient levels of sex hormones and are at risk of low levels of oestrogen. Low levels can lead to menstruation and fertility issues. Oestrogen levels fall at the menopause; this is a natural transition for women which typically occurs in their late 40s or early 50s. See *Testosterone*

Offal – See *Organ Meats*

Oils to Avoid – Highly processed *seed oils* have poor *omega-3:6 ratios* and are poor quality, unhealthy fats that were introduced relatively recently as a food source. For example, sunflower oil can have an omega-3:6 ratio of 1:200. Examples of oils to avoid include canola oil, corn oil, margarine, sunflower oil, soya oil, sunflower oil, and all generic *vegetable oils*.

Oily Fish – Fish that provide good sources of *vitamin D* and anti-inflammatory *omega-3* oils. Examples of oily fish include sardines, salmon, mackerel, anchovies, trout, and kippers.

Okinawans (Ryukyuan) – Indigenous people living on the Okinawa Islands of Japan who have one of the highest life expectancies in the world.

Olive Oil – Oil pressed from olives. Buy virgin olive oil (VOO) or extra virgin olive oil (EVOO) for a higher quality and more nutritious product.

Omega-3 – See *Essential Fatty Acids*

Omega-3:6 Ratio – See *Essential Fatty Acids*

Omega-6 – See *Essential Fatty Acids*

Organic Farming (Organic) – A method of farming that uses crop rotation and green fertilizers to maximise crop yields and nutrition. Organic farming specifically prohibits the use of synthetic fertilizers and *GMOs*. The *USDA* organic certification for produce means that the farmer used no synthetic fertilizers, chemicals, sewage sludge, or GMOs. The certification for livestock means that the animals ate organic feed, had no *antibiotics* or *growth hormones* and had access to the outdoors.

In the United Kingdom, the *Soil Association*'s definition of organic farming strictly prohibits the use of chemicals, antibiotics, ionising radiation, growth hormones, and genetic modification and requires the rotation of crops and animals to ensure healthy soil. In July 2009, the *FSA* concluded that there were 'no important differences in the nutrition content, or any additional health benefits, of organic food when compared with conventionally produced food'. However, according to the largest international research analysis ever conducted on organic foods, performed at Newcastle University and published in the *British Journal of Nutrition* in 2014, organic *fruits* and *vegetables* contain up to 69 per cent more *antioxidants* than non-*organic* crops and significantly reduced exposure to toxic *heavy metals.*

Organic Food – See *Organic Farming*

Organ Meats – Organ meats, or *offal*, are exactly what they sound like. The meat in organs such as hearts, *livers*, and *kidneys* is nutrient-rich and less expensive than muscle meat. Organ meats are high in *B vitamins*, essential *minerals* such as *iron* and *magnesium*, and *omega-3* fatty acids. Besides the more common organs mentioned, other organ meats and offal include tripe, spleen, sweetbreads (thymus and pancreas) and tongue.

Orthorexia – A term for an unclassified eating disorder, also known as *orthorexia nervosa*. Characteristics of this disorder include an unhealthy obsession with avoidance of any food that may be unhealthy. In extreme cases, orthorexia may lead to malnutrition and even death. There is evidence linking orthorexia to OCD (obsessive-compulsive disorder) because people with orthorexia demonstrate compulsive attitudes toward food.

Orthorexia can lead to social isolation and anxiety because people who have it tend to be suspicious of any food they do not consider to be pure, including foods prepared by others. While eating healthy is a good thing, taking it to this extreme is not healthy.

Osteoporosis – A disease with low *bone density* which can lead to an increased risk of fracture. It is estimated three million people in the UK have osteoporosis, and there are over 300,000 fractures every year as a result, that's one every 2 minutes. In the U.S., every 20 seconds someone breaks a bone as a result of osteoporosis with 54 million Americans living with or at risk of osteoporosis. See *Insulin Resistance*

Overweight – A term that describes an individual who weighs 10 per cent or more than the recommended healthy weight. Overweight is the point at which weight will start to have an impact on how a person looks, feels, and performs. This designation should be based on *body fat percentage*, which is a more reliable indicator of health than bodyweight. See *Obesity*

Oxalates – A kind of *antinutrient* that binds to *minerals* such as *iron, magnesium,* and *calcium* and is found in plants, nuts, and grains. Spinach contains a relatively high concentration of oxalates in comparison to other plants. Most of the iron in spinach can't be absorbed by the body because of oxalates.

P

"HEALTH IS A STATE OF COMPLETE PHYSICAL, MENTAL AND SOCIAL WELL-BEING, AND NOT MERELY THE ABSENCE OF DISEASE OR INFIRMITY."

—WORLD HEALTH ORGANISATION

Paeleolithic – See *Paleolithic*

Paleo f(x) – The world's largest Paleo health event taking place annually in Austin, Texas (U.S.). The symposium launched in March 2012 and spans over three days.

Paleo 2.0 – The term for later versions of the *Paleo diet* that, based on updated information and opinion, include foods that were not part of the original diet. These include *dairy* and starchy tubers like *potatoes*.

Paleo Alternatives – A few Paleo-friendly alternatives to common dinner favourites:

- Replace *fried potatoes* with **sweet potato** wedges. Wash and cut one medium-sized sweet potato into wedges and arrange on a baking tray. Season with black pepper, thyme, and rosemary, baste with coconut oil and then roast for around 30 minutes at 200°C / 400F / Gas mark 6.

- Replace *spaghetti* with courgette (zucchini), using two courgettes per person. Use a vegetable peeler to produce long strips of courgette, and then use a sharp knife to cut them into thin, spaghetti-like strands.

Soften the courgette for five minutes in a pan with a bit of olive oil.

* Replace *white rice* with cauliflower rice, which is a **cruciferous vegetable** that is far more nutritious than white rice. Chop a medium-sized cauliflower into florets, and then use a grater to make rice-like grains. Sauté some spring onion and two cloves of **garlic**, then add the cauliflower rice and cook for five minutes. Serves two.

* Replace *mash potato* with cauliflower mash. Chop and boil one cauliflower for 10 minutes, drain, season to taste, and mash.

* Replace *muesli* with **coconut surprise**.

Paleo Approved – a farm and ranch certification program of the Paleo Foundation.

Paleo Diet – A term coined by **Loren Cordain**. The Paleo diet (also known as the *caveman* diet or the *ancestral* diet) is a modern interpretation of what our ancestors ate in Paleolithic times (during the Stone Age) as **hunter-gatherers**. The foods at that time consisted mainly of **meats**, **fish**, **vegetables**, **nuts**, and **fruits**. It limited or excluded **sugars**, **grains**, **dairy products**, **legumes**

(beans), salt, and processed oils. ***Processed foods***, of course, were non-existent.

Researchers have found that our ancestors were lean, fit, in good health, and not plagued with modern ***lifestyle diseases*** such as cancer, ***diabetes***, and heart disease. Life expectancy was usually as good as if not better than the present day (as long as they were not being eaten by predators, suffering from poor hygiene, or contracting a life-threatening infection).

The Paleolithic era is assumed to cover more than 2.5 million years. About 10,000 years ago we entered the Neolithic era and began eating a diet that was dominated by grains. This was the genesis of agriculture, and thus, the types of food we ate began to change. With the ***Industrial Revolution*** of the eighteenth century and the advances in manufacturing and food science of the last fifty years, mass-produced food that was based on grains, sugar, and manmade substances became the norm. Unfortunately, these changes brought a corresponding deterioration in food quality as well as health.

While some prescribe to the Paleo diet based on eating the way our ancestors ate, others choose it for health reasons or **weight loss**. The basics of the Paleo diet consist of eating the following: (see also **What to Avoid**, **What to Eat**, **What to Eat in Moderation**)

- Meats
- Fish and seafood
- Eggs
- Fruits
- Vegetables
- Nuts and seeds
- Healthy fats

Paleo Fitness – An approach to **fitness** that emphasises varied natural **movement** based on our design rather than repetitive exercises and **chronic cardio**.
See **Exercise**

Paleo Food Pyramid – A method of charting preferred food ratios. The Paleo Food Pyramid differs significantly from the **USDA Food Pyramid** or the United Kingdom's **Eatwell Plate**. At the base of the Paleo Food Pyramid is animal **protein**, then **vegetables** and **fruits** in the middle, with healthy, naturally occurring *fats* at the top.

Paleo Friendly, Certified Paleo – Paleo Friendly and Certified Paleo are product certification programs for Paleo goods accredited by the Paleo Foundation.

Paleo Lifestyle – A way of approaching and living life. The objective of the Paleo lifestyle is to pick the critical aspects of Paleolithic life that make a positive difference. We do not want to turn a blind eye to the medical and technological advances that have improved human health and well-being, but integrating the best of our ancestral inheritance with the best of the present enables us to achieve optimal wellness. The Paleo lifestyle includes a focus on eating real foods, *supplementation*, exercise and activity that promotes health, quality *sleep*, effective *stress management*, maintaining good health in a *toxic* environment, developing healthy relationships, and feeling a sense of purpose. People who live a Paleo lifestyle believe that doing so will help them live healthier lives.

Paleolithic (UK: Paeleolithic) – See *About This Thing Called Paleo*

Paleo Magazine – The first and only print magazine dedicated to the *Paleo lifestyle*, first published May 2011.

Paleo on a Budget – If you have to buy or eat meat from conventional sources, buy lean cuts, trim visible fat before *cooking* and drain excess fat after cooking. This reduces ingestion of *toxins* that are stored in the animal fat. Frozen vegetables are cheaper than fresh *vegetables* and can contain as many (if not more) nutrients, as they are frozen-packed at their source. Farmers markets can also be a good source for foods direct from the supplier, which are often cheaper than supermarket alternatives. Also, buy in bulk and freeze where possible to reduce expense and wasted food.

Paleo Substitutes – See *Paleo Alternatives*

Paleo Template – The original guideline for eating *Paleo* as outlined by **Loren Cordain**. Since Dr Cordain published the original guidelines, some people have moved toward a more individualised approach. The idea is to use this Palco template as a starting point, taking into account individual goals, consider the options in terms of the health risks when we stray from this road map and to view food in the context of nutrient quality and sustenance.

Paleo Treats – Paleo-friendly snacks, desserts, and baked goods usually made with *nuts*, *dried fruit*, *coconut flour*, and *nut flours*. These treats should be rarely eaten and not as a substitute for meals.

Pantothenic Acid – See *Vitamin B5*

PAN UK (Pesticide Action Network UK) – A charity that supports safe and sustainable alternatives to hazardous pesticides. *http://www.pan-uk.org*

Parabens – A chemical preservative and additive that prevents microbe growth in cosmetic products. According to the *Environmental Working Group*, parabens, which include propylparaben and methylparaben, can be absorbed into the body, where they can cause reproductive toxicity and *endocrine disruption.* Some studies link parabens to breast cancer.

Parasympathetic Nervous System – The part of the autonomic (involuntary or unconscious) nervous system that slows the heart rate, increases the rate of digestion, gland activity and lowers blood pressure. The parasympathetic nervous system is also known as *'rest and digest'*. See *Sympathetic Nervous System, Breathing*

Parfum – A code word that can be used to describe thousands of chemicals that are used as fragrances. Because manufacturers are not required to disclose these chemicals, it is best to avoid products that contain parfum or fragrance (unless obviously identifiable as naturally sourced from essential oils) to reduce exposure to toxic chemicals and synthetic compounds such as *parabens* and *phthalates.*

Parsley – A *herb* rich in *vitamin A, vitamin C,* and micronutrients such as *iron, iodine* and *magnesium.* Improves bone health and controls blood glucose.

Passive Smoking – Smoke exhaled by a smoker plus the smoke created by the lit end of a cigarette, which can also be inhaled by a non-smoker. More than 80 per cent of second-hand smoke is invisible and odourless, and opening windows and doors when smoking indoors does not remove its effects. Residual particulate matter (including these *toxins*) builds up wherever smoking takes place—on surfaces, skin, hair, clothing, and furniture. Second-hand smoke contains more than 4,500 chemicals, including arsenic (used in rat poison) and cyanide, which is poisonous and an industrial pollutant. More than fifty of these chemicals are known carcinogens. See *Smoking, Carcinogens*

Pasteurisation – A process that heats food products to a high temperature in order to destroy harmful micro-organisms and extends the shelf life of the product (for example *coconut water* from a carton). Pasteurisation destroys some of the inherent healthy properties, and the product is less nutritious as a result.

Pastured (Pasture-Fed) – A term for animals such as cattle and sheep that have access to the outdoors and can graze pastures when grass is growing in the fields. In the winter months they are given pasture feed in the form of hay or conserved grass (silage). Meat from pastured animals is more nutritious than meat from factory-raised and grain-fed animals. For example, pastured beef is lower in total body fat, higher in *omega-3 fatty acids*, has a healthier ratio of omega-3 to omega-6 fatty acids, richer in micronutrients (such as *calcium*, *magnesium* and *potassium*) and a better *vitamin B*, and *E* profile than grain-fed beef. Organisations such as the *Pasture-Fed Livestock Association* in the UK, produce a certification mark for meat that comes from animals that have only ever eaten pasture called 'Pasture for Life'.

Pasture-Fed – See *Pastured*

Pathogen – A *micro-organism*, such as bacteria or virus, that can cause disease.

PBDEs (Polybrominated diphenyl ethers) – Man-made chemicals used as fire retardants in furniture and fabrics. Many PBDEs pose a serious risk to health, but until recently, these substances were used in a wide array of products, from electronics to bedding. Many PDBEs have been banned in the European Union and the United States because of their impact as *endocrine disruptors*, which affect both thyroid hormones and *oestrogen* signalling. Exposure to PBDEs is also linked to reduced fertility and impaired development in children.

See *Toxins*

PCBs (Polychlorinated biphenyls) – Man-made chemicals traditionally used in many products including electrical equipment, inks, adhesives, and paints. PCBs may be released into the environment, for instance, when waste that contains PCBs is burnt or stored in landfills. About 10 per cent of the PCBs ever produced remain in the environment today and can build up in animal fat. The use and production of PCBs are now banned in many countries because of the possible impact on human health and the environment, including suspected harmful effects on fertility, reproductive organs, and cancer of the liver. See *Toxins*

PCOS (Polycystic Ovary Syndrome) – A disorder of the *endocrine system* that affects women of reproductive age due to a hormone imbalance. PCOS may cause irregular or prolonged menstruation, *acne*, excessive hair growth, *obesity*, and may decrease fertility. The precise cause of PCOS is unknown, but some suspect that insulin intolerance and *inflammation* may be contributing factors. Following a *Paleo diet* reduces inflammation and may help reduce the symptoms of PCOS. Losing weight may also contribute to reducing the chances of developing complications such as *diabetes*, *high blood pressure*, and uterine cancer.

Peanuts – See *Legumes*

Perfect Health Diet – A diet outlined in a book of the same name by Paul Jaminet and Shou-Ching Jaminet. The Perfect Health diet bears some resemblance to the *Paleo diet* in that it recommends a base of *vegetables* and healthy *proteins* and eliminates *grains* and *legumes*. It differs from the Paleo diet in that it advocates a moderate amount of *safe starches* every day and allows small amounts of non-fructose sweeteners, *alcohol*, *dairy*, and *chocolate*.

Personality – A study in December 2014 at the University of California in Los Angeles (U.S.) linking personality traits to the *immune system* found that highly conscientious people had lower levels of *inflammation* while highly extroverted people had higher levels. On average, the study found the genes that trigger inflammation are 17 per cent more active in extroverts than introverts.

Pescatarian – A *vegetarian* who eats *fish*.

PFCs (Perfluorinated Chemicals) – Chemicals found in non-stick cookware, waterproof clothing, stain-proof carpets, and even dental floss. FPCs are remarkably difficult to break down and so persist in the environment for years. Human studies suggest that these chemicals may lead to thyroid disease while other research suggests them to be *endocrine disruptors* and *carcinogens*. See *Toxins*

Phthalates – Chemicals that are added to *plastics* to increase their flexibility. Phthalates are also found in a wide variety of forms such as pill coatings, printing inks, and epoxy resins that line metal cans. They are also used as fragrances in air fresheners, soaps, washing-up liquid, and even toilet paper. Phthalates have been linked to *endocrine disruption* such as early puberty in girls. High concentrations are related to low sperm count and deformities in newborns. See *Toiletries*

Physical Activity – The state of being active. Our bodies were designed to move and not just in relation to set periods of time for *exercise*. The positives of being active are well researched and documented especially in relation to health and wellbeing. Several studies suggest greater risks of early death for those who are inactive regardless of whether you are a normal weight, overweight or obese.

We should avoid prolonged sitting and hours spent being *sedentary* (which has been termed the new 'smoking') and find opportunities for *movement* whenever we can. *Walk* more, take the stairs, avoid the lifts, carry groceries home, consider a standing desk and take regular movement snacks to decrease daily non-active minutes. See *Sedentary Behaviour, Exercise, Fitness*

Physical Inactivity – See *Sedentary Behaviour, Exercise*)

Phytates – A kind of *antinutrient* most commonly found in *legumes*. Phytates bind in the digestive tract with *minerals* such as *zinc*, *iron*, *calcium*, *potassium*, and *magnesium*, making these nutrients harder to digest, which can lead to deficiencies in the body.

Phytoestrogens (UK: Phyto-oestrogens) – Are *xenoestrogens* (a class of chemicals that resemble, but are not identical to *oestrogen*) that occur naturally in plants. Some plants with high amounts of phytoestrogens include *soya beans*, whole *grains*, *flaxseeds* and *coffee*. Studies on the effect of phytoestrogens on humans are still ongoing, but there is some evidence to suggest that eating *soya* and soya products may stimulate the growth of cancer cells in women who have had breast cancer.

Phytonutrients – A substance found in certain plants such as tea, fruit, and vegetables. Evidence informs us that these plant compounds such as carotenoids and flavonoids have beneficial effects which promote good health and reduce chronic disease risk. Certain phytonutrients are better absorbed from cooked, rather than raw, food. See *antioxidants*

Pickled Foods – Often confused with *fermented foods*, however, some pickled foods are only preserved by immersion in *vinegar*, rather than through natural fermentation in brine. To ensure you are getting the additional *probiotics* and enzymes from pickled, fermented foods either purchase from a health food store that stocks such products or make some homemade fermented, pickled foods.

Plastics – A synthetic material used for a phenomenally wide range of purposes. Some plastics release substances that are toxic. Examples of this include *phthalates* and bisphenol A (*BPA*), which is a component of the packaging for thousands of food products. Research has shown that both of these compounds can leach from plastics into the foods and drinks we consume. The rate of leaching increases at higher temperatures, so imagine a plastic water bottle sitting in the sun or a plastic food container heating food in a microwave. In these cases, we are eating these *toxins* along with our food. Another example of plastic is polystyrene, which contains benzene and styrene and leaches from disposable cups and containers into warm food and drink. Polystyrene may be a *carcinogen* and may impair nervous system function. See *Toxins*

Play – An important part of the *Paleo lifestyle* that we rarely prioritise. Playful movement promotes practical strength, balance, agility, coordination, speed, skill, and mental focus. Play unlocks the mind and finds new levels of creative opportunities. Play is key to physical, mental, and social well-being, but it is often underrated and viewed as superfluous. Play is endemic to human development—a biological necessity based on our survival and one that allows us to enjoy physical activity rather than just endure it. Playful movement does not need to be complicated. Lay it out in terms of fundamental movement patterns, moves that are functional and possible to adapt for all, with challenges that can be scaled to each individual. You can piggy-back carry, or play games you enjoyed as a child such as tag; prioritise enjoyment.

Primal Play example - *http://bit.ly/FE-PrimalPlay*

Polycystic Ovary Syndrome – See *PCOS*

Polyphenols – The most abundant source of *antioxidants* in the human diet. See *Tea*

Polyunsaturated Fats – See *Fats*

Potassium – A chemical element used in tandem with sodium to regulate the volume of blood in the body and helps get rid of excess salt and excess fluids through urine. In healthy people, the ratio of sodium to potassium should be roughly 1:1. We can get the recommended 3.5 grams, the daily recommendation, by eating turkey, and fresh *fruits* and *vegetables* including pears, peaches, grapes, sweet potato and pumpkin. See *Minerals*

Potatoes – A starchy *nightshade* vegetable. White potatoes are not strictly part of the *Paleo diet.* The pros for eating potatoes are that they are nutritionally dense and contain *resistant starch,* which means that potatoes resist digestion and thus resemble soluble fibre. However, they have a very high *glycaemic index,* which contributes to *high blood sugar.* In addition, they contain *alkaloids* called *saponins,* which may contribute to *leaky gut syndrome.* People often chose sweet potatoes as a substitute for potato.

Pots and Pans – See *Utensils*

Prebiotics – Foods that pass through the gastrointestinal system undigested and support the growth of good bacteria, such as most *fruits*, **vegetables**, and *mushrooms*. Prebiotics contribute to a healthy balance of *gut flora*. See *Probiotics*

Prepared Fruit & Vegetables – Pre-washed, pre-prepared, ready-to-cook vegetables and ready-to-eat fruit sold in supermarkets. Levels of vitamins and nutrients in prepared packs of fruit and vegetables are often lower than what can be found in fresh produce. To maintain a fresh appearance salads can be pre-washed in water containing chlorine or with disinfectants such as Citrox, which is a disinfectant derived from fruit acids and used to decontaminate food. Sliced fruit can be treated with products such as NatureSeal, to prevent them from browning. For improved nutritional quality and to minimise processing intervention aim to buy packaged fruits and vegetables washed in spring water only. Better still, buy loose and unpackaged fruit and veg.

Prepared Meals – Pre-packed, pre-prepared, to-go, and ready-made meals. Avoid prepared meals, as most of them, contain lots of additives and *wheat* and/or dairy in some form and are less nutritious than freshly prepared meals. See *Ready Meals*

Price, Weston A. – See *Weston A. Price* and *Weston A. Price Foundation*

Primal Diet – A term coined by *Mark Sisson*. The Primal diet is a version of the *Paleo diet* that includes whole-fat *dairy* and reduced carbohydrate consumption and takes a more relaxed approach to other foods such as red wine, *dark chocolate*, and white rice. See *History of the Paleo Diet*

Probiotics – The name for various live bacteria and yeasts that some people take as *fermented foods* or as a dietary supplement. Taking probiotics may help keep *gut flora* in balance and alleviate symptoms of *irritable bowel syndrome,* as well as *autoimmune diseases* such as *Crohn's disease*. Probiotics may also help to maintain uterine and genital health in women. The most common forms of beneficial bacteria are *lacto acidophilus* and *bifidobacteria.* These bacteria perform the following vital tasks:

- Assist with the absorption and formation of some *B* and *K* vitamins as well as the absorption of some **minerals**
- Ferment the indigestible fibre in complex carbohydrates to produce more beneficial bacteria
- Provide protective lining of the intestines, which prevents invasion by harmful bacteria and other substances

If the gut microflora gets out of balance, then health problems may result through gut **dysbiosis**. See **Prebiotics**

Processed Foods – Any foods that are not cooked in a home kitchen. Modern food processing produces foods that are ready to eat or nearly ready to eat. They often contain high amounts of sodium, **sugar**, and preservatives and are less healthy than fresh, whole foods. Frozen fresh **vegetables** can be a healthy alternative if fresh **vegetables** are not available. However, highly processed frozen meals and packaged snack foods such as frozen pizza and candy bars are not healthy. In addition, the plastic packaging of many processed foods poses an additional health risk. See *Plastics*

Proprioception – The body's ability to detect its position in relation to its environment and to react with the proper movement. Here is a simple test for proprioception: stand with one foot in front of the other, heel to toe. Hold for thirty seconds, and then shut your eyes for thirty seconds. Repeat on the other side. See *Balance*

Protease Inhibitors – Molecules that inhibit the function of protease, a digestive enzyme. *Nuts*, especially raw nuts, contain protease inhibitors, which interfere with how the food (in this case *protein*) is broken down, and which in turn can lead to bloating and stomach cramps.

Protein – A large molecule comprising amino acids. Proteins are an essential part of the human diet because there are certain amino acids that we cannot manufacture and must get from nutritional sources. In addition, proteins contribute to satiety (*feeling full*) and may help with *weight loss*. Protein is needed for general wear and tear and to support various bodily processes, such as the *immune*, *endocrine* and digestive systems. Muscle tissues are made from proteins. These tissues break down during exercise, and, therefore, adequate supplies of protein are needed to rebuild them. It used to be thought that high levels of protein intake could damage the kidneys and bones. However, this has been disproven in healthy, exercising individuals. A recent (2007) position statement from the *International Society of Sports Nutrition* states that a protein intake of up to 2 grams per kilogram of bodyweight is both safe and desirable for active individuals.

See **Fats, Carbohydrates**

Pubmed – See **Research**

Pyridoxine – See **Vitamin B6**

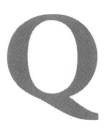

"**THE DOCTOR OF THE FUTURE WILL GIVE NO MEDICINES, BUT WILL INTEREST HIS PATIENTS IN THE CARE OF THE HUMAN FRAME, IN DIET, AND IN THE CAUSES AND PREVENTION OF DISEASE.**"

—THOMAS EDISON

QoL – See *Quality of Life*

Quality of Food – See *Nutrient Density*

Quality of Life (QoL) – A measure of the quality of a person's life as opposed to the standard of living, which addresses only money and employment. Some of the measures of quality of life include physical and mental health, education, environment, social belonging, and recreation and leisure time. See *Sarcopenia*

Quantified Self – A term for using technology, electronics, and data to gather information about the body. One example of the Quantified Self is using a biometric monitor to measure heart rate and calories burned during *exercise*.
See *Biohacking, Wearable Tech*

Quinoa – A pseudo-grain of the chenopod family. It is not recommended as part of the *Paleo diet* and should be avoided if you suffer from an autoimmune condition because of the high *saponin* and other *antinutrient* content.

R

"EVERYONE SHOULD BE HIS OWN PHYSICIAN. WE OUGHT TO ASSIST AND NOT FORCE NATURE. EAT WITH MODERATION WHAT AGREES WITH YOUR CONSTITUTION. NOTHING IS GOOD FOR THE BODY BUT WHAT WE CAN DIGEST. WHAT MEDICINE CAN PRODUCE DIGESTION? EXERCISE. WHAT WILL RECRUIT STRENGTH? SLEEP. WHAT WILL ALLEVIATE INCURABLE ILLS? PATIENCE."

—VOLTAIRE

Randomised Controlled Trial (RCT) – A

classification of scientific *research* where the population being studied are randomly assigned the treatment (test or intervention group) and the other usually a placebo or alternative treatment (control group). An RCT is known as the gold standard for clinical research. This technique is used to remove bias and to ascertain whether one treatment is more effective than the other. Randomised controlled trials are expensive and can often be sponsored by organisations that have conflicts of interest. See *Confirmation Bias*

Rapeseed Oil – See *Canola Oil*

Raw Dairy – Unpasteurised dairy products. The *dairy* products most people consume are *pasteurised.* Some people advocate drinking unpasteurized milk because they argue that the pasteurisation process kills beneficial live bacteria and enzymes. The argument against drinking unpasteurised milk is that the pasteurization process also kills potentially harmful bacteria such as *E. coli,* so unpasteurised milk may contain these bacteria.

Raw Paleo – A variation of the *Paleo diet*. The key difference is that *vegetables* and animal *proteins* are not cooked, based on the argument that heat destroys most of the nutrients. The argument against a raw diet, especially one that contains animal protein, is that raw meats and *fish* may not be safe to eat because of the presence of contaminants, and potentially harmful bacteria. Also, the process of *cooking* can increase the *bioavailability* of certain hard-to-digest nutrients by breaking down food prior to eating, in some respects, acting as the *'first stomach'*.

RCT – See *Randomised Controlled Trial*

Ready Meals (U.S. Ready-To-Heat) – A meal sold in a pre-cooked form that requires only reheating.
See *Prepared Meals*

REM Sleep – See *Sleep*

Research – The investigation and search for sound, rational explanations to establish or confirm facts. The scientific method is based on verifiable evidence and argument. However, scientists are influenced by belief and bias as to what is important, what they might and want to find, and the interpretation as to what their findings mean. There is much medical research available both online and in print, but not all of it is reliable. Although not perfect it is still by far the best way to distinguish what we believe to be true from what we know to be true. When researching, it is important to make sure that the sources are good. One thing to look for is whether the study in question is in a peer-reviewed publication. Some examples of peer-reviewed publications are the *Journal of the American Medical Association* (JAMA), the *New England Journal of Medicine*, *Lancet*, and *Science*. Another thing to consider is who provided the funding for the study. If the company financing the study has a vested interest in the outcome, you should consider that when looking at the results. If the results of a study confirm the findings of a previous study, that may also be a sign that the study is a good one.

Double-blind studies are studies where neither the researchers nor the participants know who is part of the test group and who is part of the control group. This may help to eliminate bias, as well. There are several good websites to choose when looking for information from research studies. The websites of the publications listed above are useful resources, as are websites for organisations such as the National Institute of Health and PubMed.

The strongest type of evidence and recommendation usually come from ***meta-analysis, systematic reviews*** and ***randomised controlled trials***. With ***clinical trials*** small studies produce less reliable results than large ones, so studies often need to be carried out on a large number of people before the results are considered reliable.

Other types of research include:

Anecdotal (non-scientific observations or studies), *Cross-Sectional Studies* (an observation of a study population at a specific point in time), and *Longitudinal Studies* (a series of observations of a study population over a period of time). *Epidemiological studies* (look at patterns of disease in a population and their links to factors such as diet and lifestyle). Observational studies are not the same as identifying a root cause but their findings can be useful for implementing large-scale health policy.

Resistant Starch – A kind of starch produced when foods such as *tubers* are heated and then left to cool. This process reduces the amount of glucose absorbed from the carbohydrate by the body and promotes healthy *gut flora*.

Rest and Recovery – The downtime component of a workout regime. When embarking on a new exercise regime and you start seeing great results. There is often the tendency to overdo it. One thing is for sure. High intensity workouts performed for 6-7 days a week, will result in burnout, a lack of motivation, illness and injury.

Here are five benefits of rest:

1. *Aids Recovery*: a day or two off per week of intense physical activity is required to allow bone, muscle, tendons and ligaments the time to recover and repair themselves. Muscle growth occurs during rest periods, not during exercise
2. *Keeps you healthy*: avoids the risk of the immune response being compromised due to over-training

3. *Helps you sleep*: adequate sleep allows the mind to repair itself and develop new neural connections which is useful when learning new skills

4. *Lowers stress*: decreases abnormal levels of the stress hormone cortisol. This will allow alertness, productivity and general health to be maintained

5. *More energy throughout the day*: adequate rest helps you avoid energy slumps during the day, ensuring workouts are more effective and efficient

Rest and recovery should be factored into your training regime.

Resting Heart Rate (RHR) – The number of heartbeats per minute when at rest. The normal range for healthy individuals is usually between 60 and 80 beats per minute (bpm). The resting heart rate can be an indication of your basic fitness level—in most cases, the lower, the better. The better trained your body is, the less effort and fewer beats per minute it takes your heart to pump blood to your body while at rest. Resting heart rate rises with age but can be below or above the average based on certain medical conditions. See *Hypertension*

Retinol – See *Vitamin A*

Rheumatoid Arthritis – An *autoimmune disease* that causes pain, swelling and stiffness in the joints. Typically, the body's *immune system* recognizes the cells that line the joint and does not attack them; with rheumatoid arthritis, the body's immune system attacks the cells that line your joints by mistake, causing chronic *inflammation*, making them swollen, stiff and painful. Over time this can damage the joint and surrounding tissues.

RHR – See *Resting Heart Rate*

Riboflavin – See *Vitamin B2*

Rice – A cereal grain and a staple food for a large percentage of the world's population. As a grain, rice is not part of the *Paleo diet*, although it is permitted on the *Perfect Health diet*. See *Safe Starches*

Rosemary – A *herb* which is rich in *iron, calcium*, and *vitamin B6*. Contains *anti-inflammatory* compounds, improves digestion and enhances cognitive function.

S

"HEALTH IS A LARGE WORD. IT EMBRACES NOT THE BODY ONLY, BUT THE MIND AND SPIRIT AS WELL AND NOT TODAY'S PAIN OR PLEASURE ALONE, BUT THE WHOLE BEING AND OUTLOOK OF A MAN."

—JAMES H. WEST

SAD (Seasonal Affective Disorder) – A type of *depression* that occurs at a certain time of the year, usually in the winter, due to a lack of *sunlight.* See *Vitamin D*

SAD Diet – See *Standard American Diet*

Safe Starch – A term coined by Paul Jaminet to refer to a starchy food that lacks toxins, mainly protein toxins, after normal cooking. Based on this definition safe starches would include sweet potatoes and white rice. Wheat would be a non-safe starch as it still contains problematic proteins such as gluten that remain intact after cooking. See *Perfect Health Diet*

Sage – A *herb* rich in antioxidants and nutrients such as *vitamin K.* Aids in digestion and mental disorders, such as Alzheimer's and depression.

Salad Dressings – Some very simple and healthy options include cold-pressed extra-virgin *olive oil,* organic walnut oil, and lemon juice.

Salt – Salt helps regulate the balance of fluids in the body, helps muscles to contract and relax properly, and helps to transmit nerve impulses. Salt intake was low for our hunter-gatherer ancestors, and wide-scale use of salt only began in the Neolithic period when used as a food preservative by the Chinese. Too much salt can lead to *hypertension* and may contribute to a build-up of fluids in people with congestive heart failure. Since the kidneys pass extra sodium out of the body, people with *diabetes* or other kidney problems may have difficulty regulating the amount of salt in the body. Excess salt has also been linked to accelerated loss of calcium from the bones and through the urine which can contribute to weakened bones.

Food sources of sodium include meat and seafood, beetroot, celery, spinach and carrots. Dietary sources of chloride include tomatoes, celery, olives and seaweed. If you suffer from high blood pressure, then reduce salt consumption, if you are concerned about your sodium intake get your levels checked with a sodium serum *blood test*.

If choosing to add salt to your diet, select a high quality product such as pink Himalayan salt, which is unrefined and additive-free.

San – An indigenous tribe of *hunter-gatherers* living in the Kalahari Desert in Africa. The San diet consists of foraged *vegetables* including tubers, *fruits*, ostrich eggs, and insects. Studying the San is important because it enables scientists to better understand the diets of earlier hunter-gatherers and how those diets and an active lifestyle affected their health.

Saponins – A family of *toxins* commonly found in *beans*, *potatoes*, and other *nightshade vegetables*. They bind cholesterol molecules with gut cell membranes, which increases the chance of *leaky gut syndrome*. See *Antinutrients*

Sarcopenia – A typical sign of the ageing process. Sarcopenia – meaning '*poverty of the flesh*' is characterised by loss of muscle mass, *strength*, and agility. The loss of muscle mass leads to decreased activity levels and can contribute to mobility issues, falls and fractures, *osteoporosis*, loss of physical function and *quality of* *life*. To slow or prevent the progression of sarcopenia requires the combination of nutrition, HIIT, resistance and strength training to maximise muscle mass, low-impact aerobic activities and HIIT for cardiovascular health, and balance and mobility training - to improve functionality, strength, *flexibility*, endurance, and general wellbeing.

Saturated Fats – See *Fats*

SCD – See *Specific Carbohydrate Diet*

Seaweed – A type of plant that grows in the ocean. Gram for gram, seaweed contains more *iron* than steak, as well as a high proportion of protein and *iodine*.

Second-Hand Smoke – See *Passive Smoke*

Sedentary Behaviour (Inactivity) – A type of lifestyle with little physical activity, which is defined by the *World Health Organisation* as less than 150 minutes of moderate physical activity per week. Recent research suggests that sedentary behaviour is a significant risk factor for chronic disease and mortality. Dame Sally

Davies, the chief medical officer of the UK, claimed inactivity was '*a silent killer*'.

A study of 54,000 people, published by Steven Blair, University of South Carolina, in the *British Journal of Sports Medicine*, reported that physical inactivity increased the risk of early death and were greater than the risks of smoking, diabetes, and obesity combined. Another study by a team from the University of Cambridge, recording and assessing exercise levels, waistlines and deaths of over 300,000 Europeans over 12-years, suggests that inactivity and sedentary behaviour carries a larger mortality risk than being overweight or obese.

Today, most of us are less active than previous generations and far less active than hunter-gatherer people of the past. According to *The New York Times* an Australian study found that for each additional hour of television a person sat and watched per day, the risk of premature death rose by 11 percent. Sedentary behaviour is also directly linked to back, neck and muscle pain. See ***Sitting, Exercise, Physical Activity, Movement, Sarcopenia***

Seeds – Examples include pumpkin seeds, sunflower seeds, sesame seeds, and *flaxseeds*. Avoid seed consumption if you have *autoimmune* or gut *dysbiosis* issues; otherwise, restrict seed consumption to the occasional snack, as you should be mindful of maintaining your *omega-3:6 ratio* and reducing *antinutrient* exposure. Sprouting seeds (a similar process to *sprouting grains*) can reduce the antinutrient impact. See *Seed Oils*

Seed Oils – While *seeds* in moderation are a healthy part of the *Paleo diet*, consumption of seed oils are not. Seed oils tend to be *polyunsaturated fats* with a high content of *omega-6*, which contributes to *inflammation*. See *Oils to Avoid, Trans Fats*

Selenium – An essential mineral and micronutrient. It is found in meat, fish, eggs, Brazil nuts and garlic. Selenium is thought to be required for a healthy *immune system*, offers a protective effect against some forms of cancer, and important for male fertility.

Serotonin – A *hormone* and *neurotransmitter* that impacts one's feelings and behaviour. Known as the

'*Happy hormone*'. Contrary to popular belief that serotonin is mostly made in the brain, 95 per cent of serotonin is manufactured in the gut.

Shellfish – Crustaceans, or animals that live in the ocean. Examples of shellfish include crab, crayfish, lobster, mussels, oysters, prawns, scallops, and shrimp. See *Iodine*

SIBO (Small Intestinal Bacterial Overgrowth) – A disease of the digestive system associated with gut *dysbiosis*. The symptoms of SIBO are nausea, diarrhoea, bloating, vomiting, malnutrition, and *weight loss*.

Sisson, Mark – A fitness blogger and author. Sisson has written five books about the *Primal diet* and has a primal health and lifestyle blog called *Mark's Daily Apple*.

Sitting – Prolonged periods of sustained sitting is being termed the new '*smoking*' with some experts calling it the '*pandemic of inactivity.*' A recent *meta-analysis* of 43 studies, amounting to more than 43 million people, found that significant periods of sitting were associated with a 21 per cent increased risk of lung cancer and a 24 per cent increased likelihood of colon cancer. According to Public Health England people spend nine hours on average sitting down—60 per cent of their waking time. For those working in offices 65-75 per cent of working hours are spent sitting. The dangers of prolonged sitting are a separate issue from *inactivity* alone. The use of *standing desks* and taking regular breaks to walk around the office are simple measures to mitigate the risks.

Skinny Fat (TOFI) – A term used to describe an individual with relatively low body weight and a high *body fat percentage*. A person may appear to be thin on the outside but is fat on the inside. Evidence suggests that the location of body fat, such as *visceral fat*, has more of a bearing on health than how much fat a person has. See *Overweight, Obesity*

Sleep – While sleep requirements vary from person to person, most studies suggest that adults require seven to eight hours of quality sleep a night, feeling well-rested on waking. Insufficient sleep has been linked to an increased chance of *obesity*, *diabetes*, heart disease, immune deficiency, and *depression*. Regularly sleeping less than seven hours per night can increase the risk of early death by 26 per cent and increase the risk of cardiovascular disease. Disordered sleep might lead to lower levels of *serotonin*. Scientists at Surrey University (UK) found that just one week of poor sleep can negatively disrupt hundreds of genes linked to *stress*, immunity, and *inflammation*.

Sleeping in cooler temperatures than usual (19°C) increases levels of brown fat, which uses blood sugar to maintain core temperature. This excess blood sugar could otherwise convert into body fat. Researchers have found that sound sleep in the young and middle-aged can mean better mental function in the seventh, eighth, and ninth decades when we tend to not sleep as well. Sleep deprivation reduces *leptin* and increases *ghrelin* (causing appetite to increase), reduces *serotonin* (affecting *mood*), reduces growth hormone (slowing the *metabolism* and disrupting repair mode in adults), and elevates *cortisol* (causing chronic *stress*).

See *Nap*, *Sleep Cycle*, *Sleep Tips*

Sleep Cycle – The stages of deep and non-deep *sleep* form a complete sleep cycle. Each cycle typically lasts about ninety minutes and repeats several times over the course of a night. The amount of time you spend in each stage of sleep changes as the night progresses.

The five phases of sleep are:

1. Light sleep lasting five to ten minutes
2. Bursts of rapid brain activity, body temperature drops, heart rate slows and becomes regular
3. The transition from light to deep sleep
4. Deep sleep—brain waves slow, breathing regulates, and muscles relax (the most restorative aspect of sleep, when the body repairs itself)
5. **REM** - rapid-eye movement where active brain waves cause dreaming, thought to improve the preservation of memory, learning new movement skills and enhancing problem solving ability.

Sleep Deprivation – See *Sleep*

Sleep Monitors – Devices used to track and improve sleep quality. The gold standard is to monitor electrical activity in the brain using a *polysomnogram*. Other devices measure movement (or a lack of it), breathing, and **blood pressure** during sleep. Smartphone apps are available that perform analysis of sleep quantity and quality with varying degrees of accuracy.

Sleep Tips – To improve sleep quality, try the following:

- Prioritise sleep and develop a routine, try to go to bed and wake up at the same time daily
- **Nap** no later than mid-afternoon, so it doesn't affect your sleep at night
- Avoid **caffeine** within twelve hours of bedtime
- Stop using electronic devices (smartphones, PC, tablets, TV) two hours before bedtime. The '*blue*' light emitted from these screens can suppress melatonin in the brain, making you feel more alert when it is time for bed. If you have to use your PC before bedtime, reduce the impact by downloading free software such as **f.lux**, which adjusts the light from your computer's display based on the time of day. Alternatively, wear blue blocker glasses (they usually have orange lenses to filter blue light), which reduce the impact these devices or bright evening light has on your sleep
- Avoid alcohol within three hours of bedtime. Although alcohol may make you feel drowsy, it reduces sleep quality and suppresses REM sleep, leading to less restful sleep
- Avoid food within three hours of bedtime, as the digestive process may keep you awake

- Minimise artificial bright light usage after sundown
- At bedtime, lights out and reduce ambient noise. Wear an eye mask and earplugs if that helps
- Have the room temperature between 15.5 and 21°C (60 and 70°F). Our bodies are sensitive to temperature when we sleep, especially during REM sleep. If we are too hot or too cold, we become more restless
- *Laughter* – laugh more. It reduces stress and anxiety, promoting deep, restful sleep
- Get physical activity and sunlight during the day

SLES (Sodium Laureth Sulphate [U.S. Sulfate]) – See *SLS*

Slow Food – A global movement that started in 1989 to counteract fast food and a growing disconnection with local food and traditions. *http://www.slowfood.com/*

SLS (Sodium Lauryl Sulphate [U.S. Sulfate]) – A chemical used as a foaming agent in toothpaste, shampoos, and other *cosmetics*. Research links this compound to irritation of the skin (e.g., eczema), organ toxicity, and endocrine disruption. It may also be a *carcinogen*. See *SLES, Toxins, Toiletries*

Smoking (Tobacco) – Smoking is very harmful to the human body; tobacco smoke contains many different chemicals that damage your cells' DNA. Research has shown that for every 15 cigarettes smoked there is a DNA change which could cause a cell to become cancerous. In 2008, the **World Health Organisation** named tobacco as the world's single biggest cause of preventable death. Cigarettes contain more than 7,000 chemicals, 250 of which are harmful. Of the 250 hazardous chemicals, 69 are known **carcinogens** linked to cancer of the lung, liver, bowel, ovaries, oesophagus, larynx (voice box), mouth, throat, kidney, bladder, pancreas, stomach, cervix, and some types of leukaemia. In addition to cancer, smokers have a greater risk of heart attack, stroke, COPD, emphysema, asthma, osteoporosis and other diseases.

See **Vaping, Nicotine**

Smoothies – A blended drink made from a variety of **vegetables** and **fruits**. Smoothies are packed with **vitamins** and **minerals** but can have a considerable negative impact on **blood sugar** levels because they have significantly less fibre than the whole fruit or vegetable. A smoothie can contain more sugar than a can of soft drink.

See **Fruit Juice, Juicing**

Snacks – Snacking on the *Paleo diet* is a matter of choice. It is fine to have snacks as long as they adhere to the basic Paleo principles. Make sure to consume *fruits* and *nuts* in moderation. Snacks can be a great way to get energy between meals as long as you are not eating unhealthy *processed foods* in lieu of Paleo-friendly choices. Some healthy Paleo snacks include whole fruit, nuts, and dips (baba ghanoush, guacamole, etc.) with *vegetables* or beef jerky.

Soaking – *Grains*, *nuts*, and *legumes* have traditionally been soaked overnight, which reduces mineral-binding *phytates* and enzyme inhibitors to decrease the risk of digestive issues. Soaking also helps to pre-digest the food, causing less impact to the GI tract. However, instead of trying to improve the nutrient quality of less beneficial sources of carbohydrates, focus on substituting with healthier *fruits* and *vegetables* instead. See *Sprouting*

Sodium – See *Salt, Minerals*

Soil Association – A UK charity that sets world-leading standards that exceed the requirements for organic farming in the United Kingdom, particularly for animal welfare and the use of pesticides and fertilizers. The Soil Association certifies over 80 per cent of the organic produce in the UK.

Soil Mineral Depletion – The depletion of *minerals* in soil because of poor agricultural practices. *Vegetables* today are less nutritious than in previous generations because of conventional agricultural farming practices. For example, in 1914 a cabbage had 248 milligrams of calcium and spinach had 64 milligrams of iron; in 1992, a cabbage contained 47 milligrams of calcium and spinach had 2.7 milligrams of iron.

Solanaceae – See *Nightshades*

Soup Stock – See *Bone Broth*

Soy – See *Soya*

Soya (Soy) – A protein derived from soya bean (soybean), which is a legume. As many as 60 per cent of manufactured foods contain soya. Soya can be ingested as soya flour, soya sauce or soya oil. Soya can also be used as a textured or hydrolysed vegetable protein, or as an emulsifier (*soya lecithin*). There are numerous clinical and epidemiological studies that link soya to thyroid dysfunction, digestive disorders, reproductive disorders, and cancer. Under UK government legislation, soya is classified as a major food allergen, and must be identified clearly on food ingredient labels for foods on sale, based on the European Union food labelling regulations of December 2014.

See *Legumes*

Specific Carbohydrate Diet (SCD) – A diet created by Dr Sidney Valentine Haas in the 1950s for the treatment of *irritable bowel syndrome* and *coeliac disease*. The SCD allows *vegetables*, *fruits*, some animal *proteins*, and some *dairy*. It omits grain, processed meats, and all sugars except honey and those occurring naturally in *fruit*.

Spices and Herbs – Seasonings that can be used as alternatives to salt to enhance the flavour of food. Examples include *cloves*, *rosemary*, *coriander*, *parsley*, *sage*, *mint*, *turmeric*, *thyme*, paprika, *garlic*, *black pepper*, and onions.

See *Salt*

Sprinting – A high-intensity activity and one of the most time-efficient workouts you can do, sprinting requires maximal effort. There are many benefits. It naturally produces **growth hormone**, and increases production of **testosterone** which offers incredible fat burning potential. Sprinting burns fat even hours after the workout is over, during the recovery phase. This is based on excess post-exercise oxygen consumption (EPOC), otherwise known as *afterburn*. Sprinting will strengthen your feet, ankles, calves and legs. It also improves cardio health and strengthens your heart. See *Tabata, HIIT*

Sprouted Grains – Grain seeds that have been kept moist until the plant has broken through the seed. Sprouting helps to break down or eliminate some of the things that make **grains** so difficult to digest, including **antinutrients** such as **gluten**, **phytates**, and **lectin**. However, sprouted grains are less nutritionally rich than **vegetables**, and, in general, it is better to eat them in moderation if at all. See *Soaking*

Standard American Diet (SAD) – Also known as the *Western Diet* or *Western Pattern Diet*. Typifies the diet of affluence in developed countries and is increasingly being adopted in developing countries. The SAD diet is rich in highly refined carbohydrates, high levels of dissolved sugar in the form of sweetened drinks, high levels of *salt* and artificial flavourings, poor-quality fats, and processed meats. It lacks fresh *fruits*, *fish*, *high-quality meat*, and *vegetables*. This diet is linked to everything from poor behaviour in children and *depression* to increased risks of *lifestyle diseases*.

Standing Desk – See *Standing Workstation*

Standing Workstation (Standing Desk) – An alternative to the traditional desk and chair. The computer and other work tools are on a waist-high table to enable the user to stand while working to reduce the time spent sitting on a chair. Avoid prolonged *sitting* *or* standing, alternating with intermittent periods of activity is better. See *Sedentary Behaviour*

Statins – A class of *cholesterol*-lowering drugs. While statins may decrease the chances of heart attack for a minority of people (1 in 100), they also have some serious side effects including joint and muscle aches and pain, kidney failure, cataracts, liver damage, dementia and *diabetes*.

Stevia – A herb and a sugar substitute. Stevia has no calories and does not raise *blood sugar*. However, the body may still react to the ingestion of stevia as if it were sugar and produce an *insulin* response. See *Sweeteners*

Strength – Getting stronger and gaining lean-muscle mass helps the *metabolism* run much more efficiently. Strength is linked to youthfulness, increased *bone density*, longevity, vitality, and health. Resistance exercises such as *bodyweight exercises*, weight-lifting, and strength training are excellent ways to increase strength. See *Sarcopenia, Balance, Flexibility*

Stress – The human body's response to any situation that requires change, either a physical, emotional or chemical stimulus. Chronic stress may cause problems such as *sleep disruption*, irritability, headaches, and upset stomach. Situational and acute stress may be productive since they provide the body with an adrenaline boost that may help it to achieve a goal or withstand trauma. During short bursts of stress, the *immune system* becomes more efficient at fighting infection. Recent research from the University of California, Berkeley, has shown that the brain creates new brain cells called neurons during short bouts of stress. The inability to appropriately manage the stresses of work, financial burdens, or relationship conflict has caused many to be in constant *fight-or-flight* mode.

Smartphone apps such as *Stress Check Pro* by Azumio (for iOS) measures the heartbeat to determine stress levels, and then gives calming tips to improve productivity. Playing with a pet can elevate levels of *serotonin* and dopamine, *hormones* that help to calm and relax you. *breathing techniques* can also help to restore balance by strengthening the *parasympathetic nervous system*.

Suet – Raw beef or mutton fat from around the heart and kidneys of cattle and sheep. Used to make tallow and also as a cooking fat used in many traditional British recipes. See *Tallow*, *Lard*

Sugar – There are two kinds of sugars: simple and complex. Complex sugars are those found in *fruits* and *grains* and take longer for the body to digest. Simple sugars are refined sugars such as table sugar. Eating too much simple sugar can lead to high *blood sugar*, *diabetes*, and a weakened *immune system*. A recent study published in the *Journal of the American Medical Association* concluded that eating large amounts of sugar can significantly increase the chance of developing cardiovascular disease.

The **World Health Organisation** published new guidelines in March, 2015 advising governments that adults and children should reduce their daily intake of sugars to less than five per cent of their total daily energy intake or roughly five teaspoons per day as part of their dietary guidance to reduce lifestyle disease. See *Artificial Sweeteners*

Sun Exposure – See *UV Exposure*

Sunlight – Sunshine is essential to our health. While there are a lot of warnings about the danger of too much exposure to sunlight because of the ultraviolet rays and risk of skin cancer, some sunshine is a good thing. Sunlight is a major source of *vitamin D*. A deficiency of vitamin D may contribute to an increased chance of developing breast, lung, and colon cancer. Sunshine is also an important part of maintaining our bodies' *circadian rhythms*. Exposure to sunlight helps to regulate the production of melatonin and serotonin which are required to ensure a healthy *sleep cycle*. See *SAD*

Sunscreen – A product for the skin designed to block out much of the sun's UV rays. Many mainstream sunscreens use chemical UV filters to provide sun protection. However, these ingredients such as titanium dioxide have been identified as toxic and possibly carcinogenic to humans and may be absorbed into the body through the skin. Use products that are made from naturally derived ingredients, and that include an active ingredient such as zinc oxide, which offers UVA and UVB protection. See *UV Exposure*

Supplements, supplementation – Concentrated forms of nutrition that come in a variety of forms, including pills, powders, and liquids. Nutritional supplements provide nutrients that may be deficient in your daily diet.

While nutritional supplementation is very widespread, it is better to get the nutrients you need by eating whole foods because real food is more bioavailable and likely to be utilised by the body. Food contains thousands of phytochemicals and other nutrients that work in synergy to promote good health that cannot be duplicated with a pill or cocktail of supplements.

Think food first, then plug the gaps in your diet based on advice from a health professional when deficiencies are identified, and supplementation is deemed appropriate. Some typical Paleo supplements include *fish oil*, *magnesium*, and *probiotics* to manage gut health.

Sustainability – Sustainability is how ecological systems remain productive and diverse. Some aspects of sustainability include eating a varied diet, not overfishing, maintaining healthy soil, and managing human consumption of resources.

Sweeteners – Various types of *sugars* that are added to foods, such as fructose, dextrose, sucrose, high-fructose corn syrup, maltodextrin, sorbitol, and xylitol. *Artificial* *sweeteners* also fall under this category. Better to avoid all sweeteners, including artificial.

Sweet Potatoes – A type of root tuber that has a smooth skin with colour ranging from beige, yellow, orange, red, purple, and brown. Sweet potatoes are not a member of the potato family (***nightshades***) but part of the unrelated *morning glory* family. Its flesh ranges from yellow, orange, red, brown and purple. Sweet potatoes are high in soluble fibre, beta-carotene (***vitamin A***), and ***vitamin C***. It also includes ***vitamin E***, ***vitamin B6***, and the micronutrients manganese, copper, and traces of ***potassium*** and ***iron***. They are a much better source of ***antioxidants*** than white ***potatoes*** and contain anthocyanin a colour related pigment which studies have shown to have anti-inflammatory properties.

Sympathetic Nervous System – Also known as the *fight-or-flight* system, the sympathetic nervous system is part of the autonomic (involuntary or unconscious) nervous system that accelerates the heart rate, constricts the blood vessels, and raises blood pressure. It also improves alertness and the ability to focus on the bigger picture by releasing different stress hormones, including adrenaline, to help the body deal with a threat. Prolonged activation of the sympathetic nervous system, for example by chronic stress is harmful. The *immune system* and digestion are shut down to allow more energy to be used elsewhere.

See *Parasympathetic Nervous System, Stress*

Syndrome X – See *Metabolic Syndrome, Insulin Resistance*

Systematic Review – A process to find all the relevant studies (published and unpublished), and to assess the quality of the design and implementation of each study. The objective is to present an objective, unbiased summary of existing *research*.

See *Meta Analysis, Confirmation Bias*

Systemic Inflammation – A state of long-term chronic *inflammation*, where the *immune system* is constantly on high alert. Sustained inflammation may leave one vulnerable to *lifestyle diseases*.

T

"LIFE BEGINS AS A QUEST OF THE CHILD FOR
THE MAN, AND ENDS AS A JOURNEY BY THE
MAN TO REDISCOVER THE CHILD."

—SAM EWING

Tabata Protocol – Tabata intervals are a protocol based on 20 seconds of high-intensity work, such as *sprinting*, followed by 10 seconds of rest for eight rounds (four minutes total). The Tabata protocol is a *HIIT* training method that was originally used by the Japanese Olympic speed skating team and is based on the work of scientist Izumi Tabata. The key finding from the research was that a short period (four minutes) of this high-intensity interval gave the same improvements to the aerobic system (exercise using oxygen for energy consumption) as 60 minutes of moderate-intensity exercise. The other key difference was an increase in the anaerobic system ability (exercise capability at the highest intensity without oxygen for energy use). The anaerobic system was not improved at all with moderate-intensity exercise. Tabata example - *http://bit.ly/FE-Tabata*

Tallow – Rendered beef or mutton fat. Tallow is mostly saturated fat (50 per cent) and monounsaturated fat (41 per cent). It is solid at room temperature, very heat-resistant, and a good choice for cooking, especially frying. Make sure to buy tallow from *grass-fed* animals as commercial tallow can contain fat derived from other animals or even from plant sources such as palm oil and rice flour.

See *Suet*, *Lard*

Tanning Beds – See *UV Exposure*, *Sunlight*

Tannins – Compounds found in black *tea*, red wine and *coffee* which can block the body's ability to absorb *iron*, and reduce protein digestibility. Drinking black tea or coffee with a meal, or up to an hour after, can reduce iron absorption by 60 per cent because of tannins. Drink black tea or coffee outside of meal times to prevent any potential impediment to iron absorption, other options are to drink green and white teas which contain little to no tannins. See *Antinutrients*

Tapioca – A starchy food made from cassava roots. Tapioca is gluten free but has very little nutritional value. Some Paleo recipes use tapioca flour as a substitute for wheat flour. See *Coconut Flour*

Tea, Green Tea – A (usually) hot drink made by steeping various herbs or leaves from the tea plant.

Drinking tea can be very beneficial. According to a Chinese proverb, "*It is better to drink green tea than to take medicine.*" Green tea contains much less **caffeine** than coffee. It also includes a whole host of **antioxidants** called phenols, including catechin **polyphenols**, an antioxidant that raises resting **metabolism** by four to eight per cent more than does coffee or **water.** (Catechin is the bitter taste of tea and is a **phytonutrient.**)

Green tea is especially high in a flavonoid called '*EGCG*' (epigallocatechin gallate), which may help fight cancer and heart disease. It has also been shown to reduce cancer risk, reduce LDL '*bad*' cholesterol, reduce **high blood pressure** and **blood sugar,** promote fat burning, reduce **inflammation**, preserve **bone density** and fight tooth decay, relieve **stress** and anxiety, and neutralise free radicals that cause cell and skin damage. Restrict green tea to a morning drink to avoid any detrimental impact on **sleep.** Drink black tea outside mealtime to prevent any potential impediment to **iron** absorption because of **tannins.** The longer tea leaves or a tea bag are left in water, the greater quantity the released antioxidants. A five-minute infusion compared to a one-minute brew can provide 60 per cent more antioxidants in the blood.

- Green tea is picked, rolled, and dried before the leaves go brown, giving it a distinctive aroma.
- White tea comes from the buds of the plant. They are steamed and left to dry naturally, resulting in a sweeter taste.
- Oolong tea is allowed to semi-ferment, which gives it a fruity taste.
- Black tea is made by fermenting the leaves for a few hours before heating and oxidising them, which gives it the strongest flavour and colour of all the teas.

For optimal flavour and benefits, brew at specific temperatures for the particular tea:

- Green and herbal teas – 80°C
- White tea – 85°C
- Oolong tea – 90°C
- Black tea – 100°C

Testosterone – A hormone related to muscle mass and sex drive. Testosterone is the primary sex hormone in males, but women have testosterone too, about one-tenth that of men. Testosterone regulates sexual development, libido, bone and muscle mass in men and women, and sperm count in men. Saturated fat contains ***cholesterol,***

which the body converts to steroid *hormones* including testosterone. Studies show that higher fat and cholesterol consumption results in higher testosterone levels, so those who eat low-fat diets typically have lower testosterone levels. Testosterone levels in men decline one per cent a year after the age of 30. See *Oestrogen*

Thiamine (or Thiamin) – See *Vitamin B1*

Thyme – A *herb* rich in *vitamin A* and *vitamin C* and also contains *iron*, *magnesium* and *calcium*. Contains antifungal and antibacterial compounds, and can be used for coughs when infused in water as a tea.

Tobacco – See *Smoking*

TOFI (**T**hin on the **O**utside **F**at on the **I**nside) – See *Skinny Fat*

Toiletries – Products designed to apply to the face and body to enhance the appearance or hide flaws. The skin is the body's largest organ, and whatever is put on it can enter the bloodstream. When buying cosmetics, look for companies that make organic, pH-balanced, hypoallergenic, biodegradable, eco-friendly products from businesses that make it a priority not to include harmful substances. These products are often available online or from reputable health stores. If you feel up to it, you make them yourself. In general, the fewer ingredients used in a product, the better. Read labels, and avoid *SLS*, *parabens*, *phthalates*, *parfum*, and propylene glycol, as well as petrochemicals such as petrolatum, coal tar, and mineral oil. Choose products with no synthetic fragrances, artificial colours, or preservatives. A great resource for information on what is safe can be found at *http://www.ewg.org/skindeep/* and *http://www.safecosmetics.org*

Toxins, toxicity – Any substance that can be harmful if ingested, inhaled or absorbed through the skin. Some common food toxins include *aflatoxins*, *mycotoxins*, *lectins*, *saponins*, and *phytates*. Environmental toxins include *PCBs*, pesticides, fertilisers, and fire-resistant fabrics such as *PBDEs*. Some nutrients may be toxic for certain people, so for someone with *leaky gut syndrome* or *coeliac disease*, *gluten* is a toxin. Examples of toxins in *toiletries* include *parabens* and *sodium lauryl sulphate* (SLS), which may cause irritation and *neurotoxicity*, among other things. Plastic water bottles can contain *phthalates* or *BPA*, which can leach into the beverage and have a harmful impact on health. DEET is a product used in insect repellent and is a suspected carcinogenic that is absorbed when applied to the skin or inhaled when sprayed. *Pyrethroids* are toxins that are inhaled from plug-in vapour mosquito repellents and can harm the nervous system. See *Triclosan, Heavy Metals*

Trans Fats – Fats that are uncommon in nature but are manufactured on a large scale as hydrogenated or partially hydrogenated fats. Trans fats are made by hydrogenating (adding hydrogen molecules) *vegetable oils* to make them more stable. These fats are not recognized by the body, and the body is not able to metabolise and utilise them, which can result in oxidation. Trans fats are found in foods such as margarine and some vegetable oils. They are potentially carcinogenic and should be avoided. See *Fats*

TreadDesk (Moving Standing Desk) – A product that combines a traditional desk with a treadmill to increase activity levels while working in an office environment. It is possible to use TreadDesk while seated in a chair, standing at the desk, or when *walking* slowly on the treadmill. See *Sedentary Behaviour*

Triclosan – An antimicrobial added to many products including soaps, toothpaste, and *cosmetics*. Triclosan is suspected to be an *endocrine disruptor* and a contributor to *antibiotic resistance*. A number of manufacturers, including Johnson & Johnson and Procter & Gamble, have decided to eliminate the ingredient from their products.
See *Toxins*

Triglycerides – Fat molecules that come primarily from the liver and are used for energy in the body. *Lifestyle* is one of the most common causes of elevated triglycerides, and high triglycerides are an indication that an underlying health issue, such as insulin resistance or heart disease, may be occurring. Too many *grains*, *sugars*, refined carbohydrates, and a sedentary lifestyle are major sources of triglycerides, where the liver converts excess carbohydrates into triglyceride for storage.
See *Cholesterol*

Tryptophan – An essential amino acid found in foods such as *cashews*, *walnuts*, turkey, and *eggs*. The body turns tryptophan into *serotonin*, which is a major contributor to good *mood* and healthy *sleep*.

Tubers – An underground root that stores nutrients to help a plant survive the winter and is also capable of producing new plants. Examples of tubers include *potatoes*, *yams*, sweet *potatoes*, parsnips, and turnips, as well as root *vegetables* such as carrots and beets.

Turmeric – A yellow Indian *spice* powder that is often added to curries. Topically, turmeric is used as an antiseptic and to promote healing and reduce *inflammation* such as swelling. It has also been demonstrated to have pain-relieving components.

Type I Diabetes – See *Diabetes*

Type II Diabetes – See *Diabetes*

U

"EVEN WHEN ALL IS KNOWN, THE CARE OF A
MAN IS NOT YET COMPLETE, BECAUSE EATING
ALONE WILL NOT KEEP A MAN WELL; HE MUST
ALSO TAKE EXERCISE. FOR FOOD AND
EXERCISE, WHILE POSSESSING OPPOSITE
QUALITIES, YET WORK TOGETHER TO PRODUCE
HEALTH."

—HIPPOCRATES

Ultraviolet Exposure – (see *UV Exposure*)

USDA (United States Department of Agriculture) – An organisation responsible for United States policies regarding agriculture, farming, food, and forestry. The USDA's duties include food safety and inspection, farm regulations, and protection of natural resources. While it is responsible for food safety, some have criticized the USDA for approving *GMOs* like *Monsanto's* 'ready crops'.

USDA Food Pyramid – A food guideline issued by the *USDA*. The base of the pyramid is *grains* and cereals, followed by *fruits* and *vegetables*, smaller amounts of meats and *dairy*, and tiny amounts of *fats* and sweets. These suggestions are very different from those found in the *Paleo Food Pyramid*. See *Eatwell Plate*

Utensils – To reduce toxicity for cooking utensils, minimise or avoid the use of *plastic*. Instead, use glass, stainless steel, or 100 per cent food-grade silicone for storage. Use wooden spoons and spatulas for food preparation. Use ceramic or cast-iron pans for cooking instead of pans with non-stick coatings, which can release toxic fumes at high temperatures. See *Toxins*

UV Exposure (Ultraviolet Exposure) – Conventional wisdom informs us that we should avoid the sun at all costs. However, *sunlight* stimulates the production of *vitamin D* through UV exposure, especially in the UV-B rays and can be used to treat several diseases, including rickets, psoriasis, eczema, and jaundice. The *vitamin D* that comes from sunlight may help prevent some cancers. However, prolonged UV exposure may also contribute to skin cancers. What a safe limit is for one person may be unsafe for another, depending on skin tone and family history.

Most experts recommend wearing some *sunscreen* protection if you will be exposed to the sun for a prolonged period, however the *World Health Organisation* suggest that limited exposure to UV would generate a substantial burden of disease through vitamin D deficiency.

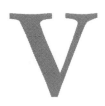

"Sleep is that golden chain that ties health and our bodies together."

—THOMAS DEKKER

Vaccinations – There is a lot of debate and controversy about vaccination efficacy and safety. The pros are that vaccines help prevent pandemics and promote human health. The cons are that vaccines may actually be harmful to the *immune system* or contain additives that are not healthy, such as thiomersal (a *mercury*-containing compound) used in multi-dose vials to prevent the growth of bacteria or fungi in the vaccine.

The World Health Organisation stated in 2006 that there is currently no evidence of mercury contained in vaccines causing toxicity because the form of mercury (*ethyl mercury*) does not accumulate, is metabolised and removed quickly from the body, unlike the most common form of mercury compound *methyl mercury* which accumulates in the body and remains there for a long time. Thiomersal is no longer used in the United Kingdom for routine vaccines given to babies and young children.

Vaping – the term used to describe e-cigarettes that use small amounts of nicotine mixed with a liquid which is vapourised to leave users inhaling a mist of nicotine instead of smoke. When users breathe out, they produce a white smoke-like vapour which is mainly water. There is some evidence that vaping can help smokers quit, and it appears to be less unhealthy than smoking cigarettes because they do not contain tar. However, **carcinogenic** compounds can still be detected in trace quantities, and some medical tests have suggested that high doses of e-cigarette vapour can suppress the **immune system** and be a possible contributory factor to cancer. See **Smoking**

Vegan – A person who consumes no animal products of any kind. This means that in addition to not eating meat, poultry, or fish, a vegan consumes no **eggs**, **dairy**, **gelatine**, or any other product derived wholly or in part from animals such as honey. None of the foods that constitute the vegan diet can provide for the daily requirement of **vitamin B12** or **vitamin D**. Because of this, vegans can face vitamin B12 deficiency. Vitamin D deficiency can also be an issue due to inadequate food sources unless there is sufficient exposure to **sunlight**. See **Vegetarian**

Vegetable Oil – An oil that is extracted from plants and is high in omega-6. Most people eat an unhealthy balance of *omega-3* to *omega-6*, so vegetable oils should be avoided.

See *Oils to Avoid, Trans Fats, Seed Oils*

Vegetables – Eat organic and in-season produce as often as possible, including asparagus, artichokes, Brussels sprouts, broccoli, cauliflower, cabbage, lettuce, carrots, celery, cucumbers, *garlic*, lettuce, mushrooms, onions, pumpkin, turnips, radishes, watercress, and *leafy greens*. See *Paleo on a Budget*

Vegetarian – A vegetarian is someone who consumes no meat (meat, poultry, or fish). Some vegetarians do consume animal products such as eggs and *dairy* products. An *ovo-vegetarian* avoids meat, fish, and dairy products but consumes eggs. With a *lacto-ovo-vegetarian*, meat and fish are forbidden, but eggs and dairy products are permitted. A *lacto-vegetarian* permits dairy products. Two vitamins that are essential for optimal health are derived only from animal products: *vitamin B12* and *vitamin D*. Vegetarians can have a hard time getting either of these vitamins through diet alone. See *Vegan*, *Pescatarian*

Vinegar – An acidic, sour-tasting liquid that has a wide variety of uses in food preparation (such as pickled vegetables) and as a cleaning product. If you use vinegar, apple cider vinegar is an excellent choice, especially if it is prepared in its traditional *probiotic* and unpasteurised form. However vinegar should be avoided for those on a low-histamine diet, or those who are strict when it comes to gluten-free produce as vinegar may be contaminated with *gluten* during the distillation process or have wheat used as part of the fermentation process.

Virgin/Extra Virgin Oil – Oils produced by the use of mechanical means only, with no chemical treatment. The term '*extra*' may denote even higher-quality oil, such as hand-pressed oil.

Visceral Fat – A type of internal fat that surrounds the vital organs, such as the liver and kidneys. Visceral fat in itself is not harmful, but an excess of it is. In one of its most dangerous forms, it can lead to excess *epicardial* fat, which surrounds the heart. See *Skinny Fat*

Vitamin A – An umbrella term for several compounds, including retinol and retinoic acid, that we get from our diet. Vitamin A helps maintain healthy teeth, skin, and skeletal tissue, as well as supporting good vision. *Oily fish* and liver are excellent sources of vitamin A., other sources include poultry and meat.

Vegetables that contain a high quantity of vitamin A include orange and yellow *fruits* and *vegetables*, including carrots, sweet potatoes, cantaloupe, and apricots. Forms such as beta-carotene, which is the orange pigment in many foods, gets converted into vitamin A in the body. A carrot meets the daily need of 0.7 to 0.9 milligrams. Vitamin A is a *fat-soluble vitamin*.

Vitamin B – There are several forms of B vitamins. They help the body regulate the energy it takes from the food we eat and also help to form red blood cells. We can easily get all the B vitamins we need from our diet. *Vegetarians* and vegans are the exceptions, as *B12* is found naturally only in meat, *eggs*, and *dairy* products. B vitamins are *water-soluble*.

Vitamin B1 (Thiamine) – Aids muscle and nerve function. Vitamin B1 is found in *eggs*, *organ meats*, *leafy green vegetables*, *nuts*, and berries.

Vitamin B2 (Riboflavin) – Keeps skin, eyes, and the nervous system healthy. Responsible for energy production. Vitamin B2 is found in *eggs*, mushrooms, *dairy*, meat, *liver*, and *dark green vegetables*.

Vitamin B3 (Niacin) – Maintains the nervous and digestive systems. Vitamin B3 is found in eggs, broccoli, carrots, avocados, *sweet potatoes*, chicken, salmon, tuna, liver, and *nuts*.

Vitamin B5 (Pantothenic Acid) – Plays a role in the metabolism of *fats*, carbohydrates, and proteins and is needed for normal growth and development. Vitamin B5 is found in *eggs*, tomatoes, and meat.

Vitamin B6 (Pyridoxine) – Aids the production of red blood cells and helps the body to absorb and metabolise amino acids and *fats*. Find vitamin B6 in *fish*, *liver*, spinach, avocados, and bananas.

Vitamin B7 (Biotin) – Helps to make *hormones*, from fatty acids, and assist in the release of energy from carbohydrates. Food sources of vitamin B7 include eggs, bananas, *organ meats*, *nuts*, and *dairy*.

Vitamin B9 (Folate, Folic Acid) – Critical to the production and repair of DNA. Vitamin B9 also helps the body form red blood cells. Good food sources include *leafy green vegetables*, salmon, *nuts*, and *organ meats*. Women also often take vitamin B9 in the form of folic acid as a supplement before conception and in early pregnancy to reduce the occurrence of birth defects such as spina bifida.

Folic acid is the synthetic form of vitamin B9 and is added through mandatory fortification to certain foods (usually grains) in many countries around the world including Australia, Canada and the U.S. As of April 2015, no European Union country has mandated folic acid fortification.

Vitamin B12 (Cobalamin) – Vitamin B12 plays a crucial role in the formation of red blood cells and the functioning of the brain and nervous system. Food sources include *fish, meat, liver, eggs,* poultry, and *dairy.*

Vitamin C – An *antioxidant.* Vitamin C helps the body to heal, to absorb *iron* and is important for the health of skin, connective tissues, and bones. According to recent research, Vitamin C may protect against immune system deficiencies, reduce cardiovascular disease, cancer, and inflammation. Good sources of vitamin C include citrus fruits, sweet potato, broccoli, tomatoes, red and green sweet (bell) peppers, and dark *leafy greens.* Current research states vitamin C does not prevent the common cold, but if you have already caught a cold, taking daily vitamin C may reduce the cold's severity and duration. Vitamin C is a *water-soluble vitamin.*

Vitamin D – Strictly speaking a hormone rather than a vitamin, it works to regulate *calcium* and phosphorus in the human body and helps keep bones strong. Vitamin D deficiency is increasingly common, especially in very young children, the elderly, and people who live in the northern hemisphere. Deficiency can lead to brittle bones, *osteoporosis,* and the bone disorder called rickets.

Deficiency has also been linked to an increased risk of *autoimmune diseases*, greater susceptibility to bacterial and viral infections, increased cancer risk, depression and increased *systemic inflammation*.

A recent study found that people with very low vitamin D are at 57 per cent greater risk of death from all causes compared with individuals with the highest levels of vitamin D. In the summer, light-skinned people can get more than enough vitamin D with ten to fifteen minutes of sun exposure wearing minimal clothing. Darker-skinned people need about forty to fifty minutes. Skin that is exposed to sunlight through a window will not produce vitamin D. Cloudy days, and shade also cut down on the amount of vitamin D the skin makes.

If you live north of San Francisco, California, or south of Melbourne, Australia, then you will not get adequate exposure during winter so *supplements* may be in order. There are two forms of vitamin D in supplement form, vitamin D2 (*ergocalciferol*) and vitamin D3 (*cholecalciferol*). D3 is the form that is produced by our skin when exposed to sunlight, and overwhelming evidence suggests that D3 has better bioavailability and more readily converted to the active form of vitamin D than D2. However, too much vitamin D can cause calcium to build up in the blood, which can result in kidney problems so knowing your levels before supplementation is important.

Good dietary sources of vitamin D include **eggs**, **oily fish** such as salmon, mackerel, anchovies, and kippers, one of the best sources. A free smartphone app that can help with tracking vitamin D from the sun is called *D Minder.*

See **Blood Work**

Vitamin D2 (ergocalciferol) – See **Vitamin D**

Vitamin D3 (cholecalciferol) – See **Vitamin D**

Vitamin E – An **antioxidant** that helps boost **metabolism** and maintain the **immune system**. Good sources of vitamin E include **nuts** and **leafy greens**.

Vitamin K – Manufactures proteins that help build strong bones and tissues and promote blood clotting. Vitamin K comes in two forms: K1, found in **leafy green vegetables**, and K2, synthesised by bacteria in the gut.

Good dietary sources of vitamin K include berries, dark *leafy greens* and *sage*. A single serving of broccoli provides our daily requirement.

Vitamins – Vitamins are classified as either *fat-soluble* (*vitamin A, vitamin D, vitamin E,* and *vitamin K*) or *water-soluble* (the *B vitamins* and *vitamin C*). The first vitamin was discovered in 1911 by Polish chemist Casimir Funk when he isolated a chemical from rice bran and showed that it could prevent beriberi. This led to similar discoveries with compounds that prevent scurvy (*vitamin C*) and rickets (*vitamin D*).

Today science recognises around a dozen essential vitamins, a group of compounds that are necessary for human health and that the body cannot produce in sufficient quantities without food (with the exception of *vitamin D*, which we make through the action of *sunlight* on the skin). It is estimated that about half the U.S. population take some form of supplement daily while nearly a third of people in the UK do the same. Be aware of synthetic versions or foods fortified with man-made versions of natural vitamins. For example, ascorbic acid is artificial vitamin C and is usually synthesised from *GMO* corn or rice starch. Artificial vitamin E can be derived from petrol, and coal tar is commonly used as the foundation for vitamin B1 supplements.

VLDL (Very-Low-Density Lipoprotein) – See *Cholesterol, Blood Work*

VOO (Virgin Olive Oil) – See *Olive Oil*

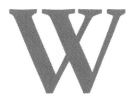

"HUMAN BEHAVIOUR FLOWS FROM THREE MAIN SOURCES: DESIRE, EMOTION, AND KNOWLEDGE."

—PLATO

Wahls, Terry, MD – Clinical professor of medicine at the University of Iowa and author of *The Wahls Protocol*, a book on how Dr. Wahls beat progressive *multiple sclerosis* using the *Paleo lifestyle*.

Waist Circumference – The measurement around the waist. People who carry fat mainly around the waist are more likely to develop health problems than people who carry fat primarily in the hips and thighs. This is true even if their *BMI* falls within the normal range. Women with a waist measurement of 35 inches (89 cm) or more and men with a waist measurement of 40 inches (100cm) or more may have a higher disease risk than people with smaller waist measurements because of where their fat lies. Breathe out naturally and measure the waist just below the belly button.

Waist Measurement – See *Waist Circumference*

Walking – Our ancestors spent a lot of time walking, an activity that is often overlooked today. Research has shown that walking:

- reduces the risk of *lifestyle diseases* such as coronary heart disease, stroke, and *type II diabetes*
- reduces the risk of *hypertension* (high blood pressure)
- reduces high *cholesterol*
- helps to prevent *osteoporosis* by increasing *bone density*
- enhances mental well-being (reduces *depression*, anxiety, and cortisol levels)
- relieves osteoarthritis
- reduces mortality rates for both younger and older adults
- reduces the risk of senile dementia

The ideal cumulative weekly walking distance was found to be between six and nine miles (9.5 to 14.5 kilometres), with no significant improvement gained by walking any further. At about one mile a day, this total distance is relatively easy to cover within a week when you consider taking the stairs, walking to local shops, and just spending more time on your feet. Some research states that aiming for 10,000 steps a day (around 5 miles/8 kilometres) is beneficial for health. Research from Wakayama Medical College (Japan) found reaching this target reduced blood pressure for those suffering from mild hypertension, irrespective or exercise intensity or duration, while work from Ball State University (U.S.) saw a drop in **waist circumference** and a loss of almost two per cent body fat in 36 weeks in overweight adults.

To track your walk progress use a pedometer (or even an app on your smartphone such as *Argus*) to keep track of your daily mileage.

Walnuts – A nut that provides good doses of **omega-3** and linolenic acid, as well as high total levels of **monounsaturated fats** and polyunsaturated fats. Walnuts have a 1:4 **omega-3** to **omega-6** ratio. Studies on overweight Americans have shown that walnuts have a beneficial effect on cardiovascular disease, which may be because of its combination of **magnesium**, **potassium**, and **calcium**.

Water – The body's most **essential nutrient**, making up a significant proportion of total body weight. Water helps flush **toxins** from the body and is required for all other nutrients, chemicals, and bodily processes to travel around and interact with the body. See **Beverages**

Water-Soluble Vitamins – Vitamins such as *vitamin C* and *B* are water-soluble and are not stored in the body. We urinate any excess water-soluble vitamins every day. Toxic overload is rare, and we need to consume these vitamins from our food daily. Water-soluble vitamins can be easily destroyed by heat or exposure to air and must be continuously supplied in the diet to maintain healthy levels. See *Fat-Soluble Vitamins*

Wearable Tech – Technology, such as watches and heart monitors that are worn on the body to measure certain functions. Born out of the *quantified self* movement, the wearable tech sector is booming, with some of the most popular devices being smart phones, smart watches, and fitness bands that measure heart rate, sleep patterns, and activity levels. Health and fitness trackers account for roughly 40 per cent of the wearables market. Advanced devices include smart insoles, which give a live update on running performance, foot strike, and gait. Some health trackers use bodily fluids to track levels of *testosterone* and other key biomarkers. Other wearables track the motion of your limbs to correct form and calculate weight progressions. There are t-shirts and vests that read your heart and breathing rates using sensors embedded in the fabric, and wireless headphones that track movement, speed, oxygen levels, and energy consumption.

Weight Loss – The net loss of body weight. For example, a decrease from 68 kilograms (10 stone 10 pounds/150 pounds) to 63 kilograms (9 Stone 13 pounds/139 pounds) is a five kilogram (11 pound) weight loss. The loss of body weight doesn't take into account whether it is water loss, fat loss or lean body mass reduction, so body fat percentage and measurements such as waist circumference are other useful metrics to better track your body composition efforts. See *Fat Loss*, *Body Fat Percentage*, *Waist Circumference*

Western Pattern Diet (WPD) – See *Standard American Diet*

Weston A. Price – A dentist and nutritionist who first proposed a link between dental health and diet. Dr Price wrote a book called *Nutrition and Physical Degeneration*, in which he concluded that some staples of the *Western Diet*, including *sugar*, flour, and *vegetable oils*, were detrimental to human health. He studied non-industrialised groups of people to make his conclusions about nutrition. See *History of the Paleo Diet*

Weston A. Price Foundation (WAPF) – A non-profit organization dedicated to continuing the work of *Weston A. Price*. The Foundation promotes good health through eating natural, whole foods.

What is Paleo? – See *About This Thing Called Paleo*

What to Eat – Here is a short list of foods to use as the basis of a Paleo approach to eating. This list is by no means exhaustive but will give you an idea of the tasty foods available to you. Try to source foods locally and find out where they come from and how they are produced. These foods will be fresher and more nutritious. The shorter distance our foods travel, the better.

- *Meats*: Eat organic, preferably grass-fed or *pastured* meats such as beef and lamb. Also eat game such as buffalo and venison as well as organic *organ meats* (liver, kidneys, etc.), but only buy from trusted sources such as farmers' markets. Make stock from leftover bones. The higher price for these high-quality meats is worth it. *Grass-fed* meats have a better ratio of *omega-3* to *omega-6 polyunsaturated fats* than *grain-fed* meats, and organic *free-range* meats are less likely to be fed *growth hormones* and *antibiotics*.

- *Eggs*: Eat eggs preferably from *pastured* chickens.
- *Poultry*: Eat only pastured, organic *free-range* chicken, duck, and turkey when possible.
- *Fish and Seafood*: Eat wild-caught varieties, including anchovies, hake, trout, salmon, sardines, cod, mackerel, and trout; farmed variants are less nutritious.
- *Vegetables*: Eat organic and in-season produce including aubergine (eggplant), kale, asparagus, artichokes, Brussels sprouts, broccoli, cauliflower, cabbage, lettuce, carrots, celery, cucumbers, *garlic*, lettuce, spinach, mushrooms, onions, turnips, watercress, and *leafy greens*.
- *Nuts*: Eat *almonds*, *Brazil nuts*, *walnuts*, chestnuts, hazelnuts, pecans, macadamia nuts, and so on. Remember, peanuts are *legumes*, not nuts, and should be avoided.
- *Fruits*: Eat avocados, apples, olives, apricots, coconuts, dates, berries, citrus fruits, peaches, pears, grapes, melon, kiwi fruit, and so on.
- Beverages: water, *coconut water*, green, white, and herbal teas.
- *Oil For Dressing*: Extra-virgin olive oil, walnut oil or macadamia oil.
- *Oil For Cooking*: Cook with extra-virgin or virgin coconut oil and avocado oil (try to avoid excessively high temperatures, and cook slowly). Also consider

suet, beef or mutton tallow, duck fat, or lard from quality pastured sources.

- *Additional Healthy Fats:* These include avocados, olives, coconut milk, and other coconut products.
- *Condiments/Seasonings:* **Spices and herbs** are best, such as **mint, coriander, thyme**, paprika, **garlic**, onions, and so on.

What to Avoid – Foods to avoid on the Paleo diet include **factory-raised** farm animals, **grains, legumes, dairy**, and **vegetable oils**. Those following the **autoimmune protocol** should also avoid **nuts, seeds**, and **vegetables** and **fruits** in the **nightshade** family (eggplant, tomatoes, etc.). Avoiding the following foods will make positive and detectable improvements to your health:

- *Sweeteners:* Avoid foods made with added sugar (such as fructose, dextrose, sucrose, high-fructose corn syrup, maltodextrin, and sorbitol) or artificial additives/substitutes such as aspartame; candy and sweets.
- *Grains:* Whole-grain or refined **wheat** (bread, cookies, cakes, pastry, pasta), rye, corn/maize (popcorn), oats (porridge), and all other grains, including amaranth, granola, millet, rice, quinoa, buckwheat, spelt, and chia seeds.

Milk: All **dairy** products including butter, cheese, cream, **whey**, curds, and **yoghurt**.

- **Legumes**: Beans and pulses, including **soya** (edamame beans, tofu, natto, tempeh, miso) and **peanuts** (peanut butter).

- **Potatoes**: White, red, yellow potatoes.

- *Condiments*: **Salt, vinegar, yeast**.

- *Beverages*: **Black tea, coffee, alcohol**, carbonated, sweetened (naturally or otherwise), **diet**, zero or low-calorie drinks; fruit and vegetable **juices**.

- **Prepared Meals**: Avoid all packed, pre-prepared, to-go, and ready-made meals, as most of these will contain **wheat** and/or dairy in some form and lots of additives.

- **Processed Foods**: Do you fail to recognise one or more of the ingredients on a food label without requiring a Ph.D. in chemistry, even though it is supposed to be natural? Then it is best to avoid.

- **Dried Fruit**: Apricots, mangoes, raisins, apple or other dried fruit.

- **Soya**: Soya milk, or anything containing soya products (soya yoghurts and desserts)

- **Vegetable Oils, seed oils**, *and spreads*: Sunflower oil, vegetable oils, margarine, rapeseed oil (canola oil), safflower oil, corn oil.

- *Industrialised* **Trans Fats** (hydrogenated or partially hydrogenated vegetable oils, vegetable shortening): Found in baked and fast-fried food.

- **Smoothies**: Fruit and vegetable smoothies.

- *Meal Replacement Bars:* Cereal, protein, snack, or meal replacement bars of any kind.
- *Legume or Grain Oils:* Soybean oil, Peanut oil (Ground nut oil), Corn Oil, Rice Bran Oil.

What to Eat in Moderation

Bananas and dense starchy **tubers** such as yams, sweet potatoes, and butternut squash are good options for post-workout nutrition if you are lean and active. However, limit these if you are trying to lose body fat or suffer from diseases such as **type II diabetes** or **hypertension.** **Nuts** are fine, but be careful with your quantities. They are easy to eat in significant amounts and given their high **omega-3** to **omega-6** ratios, nuts can be pro-inflammatory in large doses.

Wheat – A cereal **grain** used to make bread, cookies, cakes, pastry, pasta, and other baked goods. It is one of the foods to avoid when following the Paleo diet. Sweets, sauces, and processed foods could also contain forms of flour.

Whey – A *protein* found in *dairy* products. *Whey protein* is often sold as a nutritional **supplement** and is responsible for some milk allergies. See *Casein*

White Potatoes – See *Potatoes*

White Tea – See *Tea*

WHO – See *World Health Organization*

Whole 30 – See *Challenges*

Wild-Caught – A term that identifies fish that come from the ocean or other natural habitat as opposed to fish raised on a farm. Farmed fish eat a diet that includes corn and other things that they would not eat in the wild, and they tend to have lower levels of *omega-3* than wild-caught fish.

Wild Foods – See *Foraging*

Wild Game, Wild Meat – See *Game*

WOD (Workout of the Day) – A common *Crossfit* term. These are workouts published daily for Crossfit adherents.

Wolf, Robb – A former research student of *Loren Cordain*. Wolf wrote a bestselling book called *The Paleo Solution: The Original Human Diet*. He has a blog, a popular podcast and teaches seminars around the world on nutrition and diet. See *History of the Paleo Diet*

Workout Time – Research shows that, overall, the best time of the day to *exercise* is between 4 o'clock and 5 o'clock in the afternoon when the body temperature is at its highest. (It is at its lowest just before waking.) *Testosterone* production is highest earlier in the day, so mid-morning to early afternoon is best for strength and sprint training, where output is five per cent higher. Aerobic work is best during the mid-afternoon when endurance work is four per cent higher. Research also shows that morning exercisers are more likely to stick to it than people who exercise later in the day.

World Health Organization (WHO) – An international agency that is concerned with and highlights international public health issues. The WHO was formed in 1948.

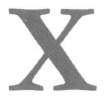

"TO KNOW WHAT YOU KNOW AND WHAT YOU DO NOT KNOW, THAT IS TRUE KNOWLEDGE."

—CONFUCIUS

Xanthan Gum (E415) – A common food additive that is used as a thickener. Xanthan gum is sometimes made from corn, *wheat*, or *soya*. Consequently, since many *gluten-free* recipes use xanthan gum as a thickener, some gluten-free foods may contain small amounts of gluten. See *E Numbers*

Xenoestrogens – Biological or synthetic compounds that mimic the effects of *oestrogen*. Some common materials that contain xenoestrogens are compounds such as *PCBs*, *BPAs*, and *phthalates*, as well as prescription oestrogen and birth control pills. Xenoestrogens are linked to problems such as early puberty in girls and reproductive problems. See *Phytoestrogens*

Xylitol – An alcohol found in plants. Xylitol is used as a sugar substitute because of its sweet flavour. It has a lower *glycaemic index* than table sugar, but it is also a *polyol* (the P in *FODMAP*) and may cause bloating and indigestion.

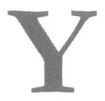

"WE ARE WHAT WE REPEATEDLY DO. EXCELLENCE, THEN, IS NOT AN ACT, BUT A HABIT."

—ARISTOTLE

Yams – A type of root *tuber* that has a thick, rough, dark brown scaly skin, the flesh is quite dry, starchy and can be quite bitter to taste. Its flesh is usually white or yellow in colour. Yams are high in soluble fibre, and *vitamin C*. This tuber is an excellent source of the *vitamin B* group, especially *vitamin B6*, and a good source of the micronutrients manganese, copper, and *potassium* with traces of phosphorous, *magnesium* and *iron*. In the U.S. and Canada, the soft sweet potato variety with deep orange flesh is commonly referred to as a yam. However, it is not a member of the *potato* or *sweet potato* family.

Yeast – A microscopic, single-cell fungus. There are two main categories of yeast: harmful and beneficial. Candida is a harmful yeast that causes yeast infections and jock itch (fungal infection of the groin). Cutting out *sugar* and *grains* from the diet may help eliminate candida. Yeast can grow in the small intestine and cause small intestinal bacterial overgrowth (*SIBO*).

The kind of yeast found in foods such as *kombucha*, *kefir*, and *fermented vegetables* is believed to be beneficial. This type of yeast can control and eliminate harmful yeast in the gut.

Nutritional yeast which is an inactive form of yeast that bakers and brewers use is regarded as neutral by some in the Paleo community and is often used as a 'cheese' substitute, however there was recent research published in January 2013 by the immunologist Dr. Aristo Vojdani, suggesting that those who are following a gluten-free diet *can* have *cross-reactivity* issues with yeast. In other words the person can suffer the same inflammatory response as if they had eaten gluten, so something to bear in mind if you are particularly sensitive to gluten.

Yoghurt (yogurt) – A *fermented* milk product. Yoghurt can be made from cow, sheep, or goat milk, although there are coconut-milk yoghurt options available for those who choose not to consume animal milk. Live yoghurt contains *probiotic* bacteria such as acidophilus. Probiotic bacteria are the good bacteria that inhabit the gut and help protect the gut lining, preventing infections.

Eating live yoghurt can help to:

- promote healthy digestion
- regulate bowel movements
- ease ***dysbiosis*** (the imbalance between good and bad bacteria in the gut)
- boost immunity
- useful in the treatment of vaginal infections

Different yoghurts contain different varieties and strains of probiotic bacteria. However, most contain either acidophilus (*lactobacillus acidophilus*) or bifidobacteria.

Z

"LEARN FROM YESTERDAY, LIVE FOR TODAY, HOPE FOR TOMORROW. THE IMPORTANT THING IS NOT TO STOP QUESTIONING."

—ALBERT EINSTEIN

Zero-Carb – A diet that includes only animal fats and proteins and entirely excludes *fruits*, *vegetables*, and other sources of carbohydrates. A zero-carb diet also includes certain kinds of *dairy* such as *ghee*.

Zinc – An important mineral that plays a vital role in cell metabolism, healing, and production of DNA. Oysters provide more zinc per serving than any other food. Too little zinc can result in a compromised *immune system* and hair loss. Some evidence suggests that once you have a cold, zinc may cut it short. Zinc supplements may also slow age-related degeneration of the centre of the retina.

Zonulin – A protein that helps to regulate the permeability of cells in the digestive tract. Faulty zonulin pathways may be a contributing factor in *leaky gut syndrome*, *diabetes*, and *autoimmune diseases*, including *coeliac disease*.

RESONANCES
RESOURCES

"A MAN WITH CONVICTION IS A HARD MAN TO CHANGE. TELL HIM YOU DISAGREE AND HE TURNS AWAY. SHOW HIM FACTS OR FIGURES AND HE QUESTIONS YOUR SOURCES. APPEAL TO LOGIC AND HE FAILS TO SEE YOUR POINT."

—LEON FESTINGER

A. Vojdani and I. Tarash, "Cross-Reaction between Gliadin and Different Food and Tissue Antigens," Food and Nutrition Sciences, Vol. 4 No. 1, 2013, pp. 20-32.

Abramson J, Wright JM. "Are lipid-lowering guidelines evidence-based?" Lancet 2007 Jan 20;369(9557):168-9. PubMed PMID: 17240267.

"Aging in motion: the facts about sarcopenia. Alliance for Aging Research website." http://www.aginginmotion.org/wp-content/uploads/2011/04/sarcopenia_fact_sheet.pdf. Updated April 2011. Accessed February 19, 2014.

"Alcohol and Depression." (n.d). Retrieved 10 March, 2015, from http://www.rcpsych.ac.uk/healthadvice/problemsdisorders/alcoholdepression.aspx.

"Alcohol's Effects on the Body." (n.d.). Retrieved September 25, 2014, from http://www.niaaa.nih.gov/alcohol-health/alcohols-effects-body.

Ahern, Amy L. et al. "A qualitative exploration of young women's attitudes towards the thin ideal," Journal of Health Psychology 16, no. 1 (January 2011): 70–79, http://www.ncbi.nlm.nih.gov/pubmed/20709877.

American Physical Therapy Association, "Private Practice Section," accessed January 28, 2014, http://www.ppsapta.org.

Anderson LA, McMillan SA, Watson RG, Monaghan P, Gavin AT, Fox C, Murray LJ: "Malignancy and mortality in a population-based cohort of patients with coeliac disease or gluten sensitivity". World J Gastroenterol 2007

Anderson JW, Reynolds R, Bush HM, Rinsky JL, Washnock C. "Effect of a behavioral/nutritional intervention program on weight loss in obese adults: A randomized controlled trial." Postgrad Med 2011

"Artificial Sweeteners. (n.d.)." Retrieved September 25, 2014, from http://www.hsph.harvard.edu/nutritionsource/healthy-drinks/artificial-sweeteners/.

Audettte, Ray "NeanderThin: Eat Like a Caveman to Achieve a Lean, Strong, Healthy Body" (St Martin's Press, 2000)

Austin GL, Thiny MT, Westman EC, Yancy WS Jr, Shaheen NJ. "A very low-carbohydrate diet improves gastroesophageal reflux and its symptoms." (2006, August 1). Retrieved September 17, 2014, from http://www.ncbi.nlm.nih.gov/pubmed/16871438?dopt=AbstractPlus.

Badrick, Ellen et al. "The relationship between alcohol consumption and cortisol secretion in an aging cohort," Journal of Clinical Endocrinology and Metabolism 93, no. 3 (March 2008): 750–57, doi: 10.1210/jc.2007-0737.

Baicy, K. et al. "Leptin replacement alters brain response to food cues in genetically leptin-deficient adults," Proceedings of the National Academy of Sciences of the United States of America, November 2007, http://www.pnas.org/content/104/46/18276.

Barnett K, Mercer SW, Norbury M, Watt G, Wyke S, Guthrie B (2012). "Epidemiology of multimorbidity and implications for health care, research, and medical education: a cross-sectional study."

Bassett, D et al. "Effects of a 10,000 steps per day goal in overweight adults.", American journal of health promotion: AJHP 11/2006; 21(2):85-9. DOI: 10.4278/0890-1171-21.2.85

Bastard, J.P. et al. "Recent advances in the relationship between obesity, inflammation, and insulin resistance," European Cytokine Network 17, no. 1 (March 2006): 4–12, http://www.ncbi.nlm.nih.gov/pubmed/16613757.

Batmanghelidj, F. "Your Body's Many Cries for Water: A Revolutionary Natural Way to Prevent Illness and Restore Good Health," 4th ed. Tagman: Falls Church, VA: 2007.

Behm DG, Chaouachi A. "A review of the acute effects of static and dynamic stretching on performance.", Eur J Appl Physiol. 2011 Nov;111(11):2633-51. doi: 10.1007/s00421-011-1879-2. Epub 2011 Mar 4.

Berto, Rita. "The Role of Nature in Coping with Psycho=Physiological Stress: A Literature Review on Restorativeness", Behav. Sci. 2014, 4(4), 394-409

Björntorp, P. "Do stress reactions cause abdominal obesity and comorbidities?" Obesity Reviews 2, no. 2, (May 2001): 73–86, http://www.ncbi.nlm.nih.gov/pubmed/12119665.

Blakey, W P. Stretching Without Pain. Canada: Twin Eagles Educational & Healing Institute, 1994, p.20.

Boers I, Muskiet FA, Berkelaar E, Schut E, Penders R, Hoenderdos K, Wichers HJ, Jong MC. "Favourable effects of consuming a Palaeolithic-type diet on characteristics of the metabolic syndrome: a randomized controlled pilot-study.", Lipids Health Dis. 2014 Oct 11

Boutcher, Stephen H. "High-intensity intermittent exercise and fat loss," Journal of Obesity, 2011, http://www.ncbi.nlm.nih.gov/pubmed/21113312.

Brandtzaeg P, Halstensen TS, Kett K, Krajci P, Kvale D, Rognum TO, Scott H, Sollid LM. "Immunobiology and immunopathology of human gut mucosa: humoral immunity and intraepithelial lymphocytes." Gastroenterology 1989, 97

British Orthopaedic Association, 2007. "The Care of Patients with Fragility Fracture". London: British Orthopaedic Association.

Brown J.E., Mosley M., Aldred S. "Intermittent fasting: A dietary intervention for prevention of diabetes and cardiovascular disease?", (2013) British Journal of Diabetes and Vascular Disease, 13 (2) , pp. 68-72.

Brown KM, Arthur JR; "Selenium, selenoproteins and human health: a review." Public Health Nutr. 2001 Apr;4(2B):593-9.

Brugts JJ, Yetgin T, Hoeks SE, Gotto AM, Shepherd J, Westendorp RG, de Craen AJ, Knopp RH, Nakamura H, Ridker P, van Domburg R, Deckers JW. "The benefits of statins in people without established cardiovascular disease but with cardiovascular risk factors: meta-analysis of randomised controlled trials." BMJ. 2009 Jun 30;338:b2376. doi: 10.1136/bmj.b2376

Bulhões, A. C. et al. "Correlation between lactose absorption and the C/T-13910 and G/A-22018 mutations of the lactase-phlorizin hydrolase (LCT) gene in adult-type hypolactasia," Brazilian Journal of Medical and Biological Research 40, no. 11 (November 2007): 1441–46, http://www.ncbi.nlm.nih.gov/pubmed/17934640.

Burks W, Helm R, Stanley S, Bannon GA, "Food allergens". Curr Opin Allergy Clin Immunol 1 (3): 243–8. (June 2001).

Calle, E. E. et al. "Body-mass index and mortality in a prospective cohort of U.S. adults," New England Journal of Medicine 341, no. 15 (October 1999):1097–105.

Calogero, Rachel M. "Objectification processes and disordered eating in British women and men," Journal of Health Psychology 14, no. 3 (April 2009): 394–402, http://www.ncbi.nlm.nih.gov/pubmed/19293301.

Catassi C1, Fabiani E, Iacono G, D'Agate C, Francavilla R, Biagi F, Volta U, Accomando S, Picarelli A, De Vitis I, Pianelli G, Gesuita R, Carle F, Mandolesi A, Bearzi I, Fasano A. "A prospective, double-blind, placebo-controlled trial to establish a safe gluten threshold for patients with celiac disease.", Am J Clin Nutr. 2007 Jan

Catassi C, Fasano A. "Celiac disease." Curr Opin Gastroenterol 2008, 24:687-691

Cesvet, Bertrand. "Conversation Capital: How to Create Stuff People Love to Talk About." Upper Saddle River, NJ: FT Press, 2008.

Chaix, Amandine et al. "Time-Restricted Feeding Is a Preventative and Therapeutic Intervention against Diverse Nutritional Challenges", Cell Metabolism , Volume 20 , Issue 6 , 991 – 1005

Chaouachi A1, Castagna C, Chtara M, Brughelli M, Turki O, Galy O, Chamari K, Behm DG. "Effect of warm-ups involving static or dynamic stretching on agility, sprinting, and jumping performance in trained individuals.", J Strength Cond Res. 2010 Aug;24(8):2001-11.

Chowdhury R, Warnakula S, Kunutsor S, Crowe F, Ward HA, Johnson L, et al. "Association of Dietary, Circulating, and Supplement Fatty Acids With Coronary Risk: A Systematic Review and Meta-analysis." Ann Intern Med. 2014;160:398-406.

Chung KT, Wong TY, Wei CI, Huang YW, Lin Y., "Tannins and Human Health: A Review," Critical Reviews in Food Science and Nutrition, Vol. 38, No. 6, pp. 421-64, Aug. 1998.

Claire E. Berryman, PhD; Sheila G. West, PhD; Jennifer A. Fleming, MS, RD; Peter L. Bordi, PhD; Penny M. Kris-Etherton, PhD, RD, "Effects of Daily Almond Consumption on Cardiometabolic Risk and Abdominal Adiposity in Healthy Adults With Elevated LDL-Cholesterol: A Randomized Controlled Trial", J Am Heart Assoc. 2015; 4: e000993 originally published January 5, 2015

Coon JT et al., "Does Participating in Physical Activity in Outdoor Natural Environments Have a Greater Effect on Physical and Mental Wellbeing than Physical Activity Indoors? A Systematic Review." Environmental Science & Technology, 2011

Cordain, L. "Cereal grains: humanity's double-edged sword," World Review of Nutrition and Dietetics 84 (1999): 19–73.

Cordain, L. et al. "Modulation of immune function by dietary lectins in rheumatoid arthritis," British Journal of Nutrition 83, no. 3 (March 2000): 207–17, http://www.ncbi.nlm.nih.gov/pubmed/10884708.

Cordain, L. et al. "Origins and evolution of the Western diet: health implications for the 21st century," American Journal of Clinical Nutrition 81, no 2 (February 2005): 341–54.

Cordain L, Eaton SB, Miller JB, Mann N, Hill K. "The paradoxical nature of hunter-gatherer diets: meat-based, yet non-atherogenic.", Eur J Clin Nutr. 2002 Mar

Cordain, Loren. "The Paleo Answer: 7 Days to Lose Weight, Feel Great, Stay Young." Hoboken, NH: John Wiley and Sons, 2012.

Cordain, Loren. "The Paleo Diet: Lose Weight and Get Healthy by Eating the Foods You Were Designed to Eat." Rev. ed. Hoboken, NJ: John Wiley & Sons: 2011.

Crabb, David W. and Suthat Liangpunsakul. "Alcohol and lipid metabolism," Journal of Gastroenterology and Hepatology 21, supplement 3 (October 2006): S56–60, http://www.ncbi.nlm.nih.gov/pubmed/16958674.

Crujeiras AB, Goyenechea E, Abete I, Lage M, Carreira MC, Martínez JA, Casanueva FF. "Weight regain after a diet-induced loss is predicted by higher baseline leptin and lower ghrelin plasma levels." J Clin Endocrinol Metab. 2010 Nov

CTT Collaborators. Efficacy and safety of cholesterol-lowering treatment: prospective meta-analysis of data from 90 056 participants in 14 randomised trials of statins. Lancet. 2005; 366: 1267-1278.

D. B. Kell, "Iron behaving badly: inappropriate iron chelation as a major contributor to the aetiology of vascular and other progressive inflammatory and degenerative diseases," BMC Med. Genomics, 2009.

D. B. Kell, "Towards a unifying, systems biology understanding of large-scale cellular death and destruction caused by poorly liganded iron: Parkinson's, Huntington's, Alzheimer's, prions, bactericides, chemical toxicology and others as examples," Arch. Toxicol., 2010, 577, 825–889.

Dalla Pellegrina, C. et al."Effects of wheat germ agglutinin on human gastrointestinal epithelium: insights from an experimental model of immune/epithelial cell interaction," Toxicology and Applied Pharmacology 237, no. 2 (June 2009): 146–53, http://www.ncbi.nlm.nih.gov/pubmed/19332085.

Daniel, Kaayla T. "The Whole Soy Story: The Dark Side of America's Favorite Health Food." Washington, DC: New Trends, 2009.

Davis, William "Wheat Belly : The effortless health and weight-loss solution - no exercise, no calorie counting, no denial" (Harper Thorsons 2015)

Davidson K.M. (1995) "Diagnosis of depression in alcohol dependence: changes in prevalence with drinking status." British Journal of Psychiatry 166: 199-204.

De Wit, B. et al. "Biomechanical analysis of the stance phase during barefoot and shod running," Journal of Biomechanics 33, no. 3 (March 2000): 269–78, http://www.ncbi.nlm.nih.gov/pubmed/10673110.

"Deaths from NDCs," accessed January 28, 2012, http://www.who.int/gho/ncd/mortality_morbidity/ncd_total/en/index.html.

"Department of Health: The Management of Adult Diabetes Services in the NHS," accessed January 28, 2013, http://www.publications.parliament.uk/pa/cm201213/cmselect/cmpubacc/289/289.pdf.

"Department of Health (2012). Report. Long-term conditions compendium of Information: 3rd edition," accessed January 14 2014

Diamond, Jared, "The Worst Mistake in the History of the Human Race," Discover, May 1987, http://discovermagazine.com/1987/may/02-the-worst-mistake-in-the-history-of-the-human-race.

Diamon, Jared "Guns, Germs, and Steel: The Fate of Human Societies" (New Vintage, 1998)

Dincer, C.; Karaoglan, M.; Erden, F.; Tetik, N.; Topuz, A.; Ozdemir, F. (2011). "Effects of Baking and Boiling on the Nutritional and Antioxidant Properties of Sweet Potato Cultivars". Plant Foods for Human Nutrition 66 (4): 341–347.

"Do You Know Some of the Health Risks of Being Overweight? (n.d.)." Retrieved September 26, 2014, from http://win.niddk.nih.gov/publications/health_risks.htm.

Drago, S. et al. "Gliadin, zonulin and gut permeability: Effects on celiac and non-celiac intestinal mucosa and intestinal cell lines," Scandinavian Journal of Gastroenterology 41, no. 4, (April 2006): 408–19, http://www.ncbi.nlm.nih.gov/pubmed/16635908.

Duntas LH; "Selenium and the thyroid: a close-knit connection." J Clin Endocrinol Metab. 2010 Dec;95(12):5180-8. Epub 2010 Sep 1.

Eades, Michael R, Eades, Mary Dan "The Protein Power Lifeplan" (Grand Central Publishing 2001)

Eaton, Konner, Shostak "The Paleolithic Prescription" (Harper Collins, 1989)

Eatwell Plate - accessed January 29, 2015, http://www.nhs.uk/Livewell/Goodfood/Pages/eatwell-plate.aspx

"Eating Disorders," National Health Services (NHS) website, accessed January 29, 2014, http://www.nhs.uk/conditions/Eating-disorders/Pages/Introduction.aspx

Eckel RH, Jakicic JM, Ard JD, de Jesus JM, Houston Miller N, Hubbard VS, et al. 2013 "AHA/ACC guideline on lifestyle management to reduce cardiovascular risk: a report of the American College of Cardiology/American Heart Association Task Force on Practice Guidelines." Circulation. 2014;129(25 Suppl 2):S76-99. PMID: 24222015

Edwards, Darryl. "Nutrition: Is a Fruit Smoothie Better Than a Can of Coke?" The Fitness Explorer, last modified November 7, 2012, http://www.thefitnessexplorer.com/home/2012/11/7/nutrition-is-a-fruit-smoothie-better-than-a-can-of-coke.html.

Edwards, Darryl. "Paleo Fitness: A Primal Training and Nutrition Program to Get Lean, Strong and Healthy" (Berkeley, CA: Ulysses Press, 2013).

"Effect of tea and other dietary factors on iron absorption." Critical Reviews in Food Science and Nutrition, Sep. 2000, Vol. 40, No. 5, pp. 371-98.

"Eggs – British Heart Foundation", British Heart Foundation website, accessed December 12, 2014, https://www.bhf.org.uk/heart-matters-magazine/nutrition/eggs. (2007)

Eliot, Lise. "What's Going on in There?: How the Brain and Mind Develop in the First Five Years of Life." New York: Bantam, 2000.

Elizabeth Lissiman, Alice L Bhasale and Mark Cohen, "Garlic for the Common Cold." Retrieved 11 November, 2014, from http://onlinelibrary.wiley.com/doi/10.1002/14651858.CD006206.pub4/full.

Elkind, David. "The Power of Play: Learning what comes naturally," American Journal of Play, 2008.

Erickson, Kirk I. et al. "Exercise Training Increases Size of Hippocampus and Improves Memory." Proceedings of the National Academy of Sciences, January 2011.

Escott-Stump S, ed. "Nutrition and Diagnosis-Related Care." 6th ed. Philadelphia, Pa: Lippincott, Williams & Wilkins; 2008.

European Food Safety Authority (website), "About EFSA", Retrieved 15 April, 2015, from http://www.efsa.europa.eu/en/aboutefsa.htm.

"F as in Fat: How Obesity Threatens America's Future 2012." Trust for America's Health, September 2012, http://www.healthyamericans.org/report/100.

Fallon, Sally, "Nourishing Traditions: The Cookbook That Challenges Politically Correct Nutrition and the Diet Dictocrats" (New Trends Publishing, 2nd Edition 2009)

Fasano, A. "Surprises from celiac disease," Scientific American (2009), accessed December 8, 2012, http://www.scientificamerican.com/article.cfm?id=celiac-disease-insights.

Feinman RD, Fine EJ: "A calorie is a calorie" violates the second law of thermodynamics. Nutr J 2004

Finkelstein, E. A. et al. "Obesity and severe obesity forecasts through 2030," American Journal of Preventive Medicine 42, no. 6 (June 2012): 563–70, http://www.ncbi.nlm.nih.gov/pubmed/22608371.

Ford ES1, Caspersen CJ. "Sedentary behaviour and cardiovascular disease: a review of prospective studies.", Int J Epidemiol. 2012 Oct;41(5):1338-53. doi: 10.1093/ije/dys078. Epub 2012 May 26.

Foster-Powell K, Holt SH, Brand-Miller JC. International table of glycemic index and glycemic load values: 2002. Am J Clin Nutr. 2002

Francis, G. et al. "The biological action of saponins in animal systems: a review," British Journal of Nutrition 88, no. 6 (December 2002): 587–605, nih.gov/pubmed/12493081.

Frassetto, L. A. et al. "Metabolic and physiologic improvements from consuming a Paleolithic, hunter-gatherer type diet," European Journal of Clinical Nutrition 63, no. 8 (February 2009): 947–55, http://www.ncbi.nlm.nih.gov/pubmed/19209185.

Fredrickson BL, Grewen KM, Coffey KA, et al. "A functional genomic perspective on human well-being." Proc Natl Acad Sci USA. 2013;110(33):13684–13689.

"Fruit and vegetable consumption and all-cause, cancer and CVD mortality: analysis of Health Survey for England data" - http://jech.bmj.com/content/early/2014/03/03/jech-2013-203500.

Garber CE et al., "American College of Sports Medicine position stand. Quantity and quality of exercise for developing and maintaining cardiorespiratory, musculoskeletal, and neuromotor fitness in apparently healthy adults: guidance for prescribing exercise." Med Sci Sports Exerc. 2011.

Gadgaudas, Nora "Primal Body, Primal Mind : The Secrets of the Paleo Diet and New Discoveries in Brain and Longevity Science" (Healing Arts Press, 2011)

Gershon, Michael D. "The Second Brain: A Groundbreaking New Understanding of Nervous Disorders of the Stomach and Intestine." New York: HarperCollins, 1999.

"Global Health Risks: Mortality and burden of disease attributable to selected major risks," World Health Organization, 2009, http://www.who.int/healthinfo/global_burden_disease/GlobalHealthRisks_report_full.pdf.

"Global status report on noncommunicable diseases 2010," last modified April 2011, http://www.who.int/nmh/publications/ncd_report2010/en.

"Global status report on noncommunicable diseases 2014," last modified January 2015, http://apps.who.int/iris/bitstream/10665/148114/1/9789241564854_eng.pdf?ua=1

"Global Vaccine Safety - Thiomersal and vaccines: questions and answers," last modified July 2006, Retrieved 18 October 2014 from http://www.who.int/vaccine_safety/committee/topics/thiomersal/questions/en/.

Grant, Tara "The Hidden Plague: A Field Guide for Surviving & Overcoming Hidradenitis Suppurativa" (Primal Blueprint Publishing 2013)

Greenfield, Ben "Beyond Training: Mastering Endurance, Health and Life" (Victory Belt, 2014)

H. Okada, C. Kuhn, H. Feillet, and J. Bach, "The 'hygiene hypothesis' for autoimmune and related disease: An update." Clin Exp Immunol. Apr 2010; 160 (1): 1–9. Retrieved Sept 25, 2014, from http://www.ncbi.nlm.nih.gov/pmc/articles/PMC2841828/.

Halfdan Petursson, Johann A Sigurdsson, Calle Bengtsson, Tom I L Nilsen, Linn Getz, "Is the use of cholesterol in mortality risk algorithms in clinical guidelines valid? Ten years prospective data from the Norwegian HUNT 2 study", J Eval Clin Pract. 2012 February; 18(1): 159–168. doi: 10.1111/j.1365-2753.2011.01767.x, http://www.ncbi.nlm.nih.gov/pmc/articles/PMC3303886/, Retrieved 8 April 2015.

Hamilton, Marc T., et al. "Too little exercise and too much sitting: Inactivity physiology and the need for new recommendations on sedentary behavior," Current Cardiovascular Risk Reports 2, no. 4 (July 2008): 292–298, http://www.ncbi.nlm.nih.gov/pmc/articles/PMC3419586.

Hamilton MT1, Hamilton DG, Zderic TW, "Role of low energy expenditure and sitting in obesity, metabolic syndrome, type 2 diabetes, and cardiovascular disease." Diabetes. 2007 Nov;56(11):2655-67. Epub 2007 Sep 7.

Han KH, Matsumoto A, Shimada K et al. "Effects of anthocyanin-rich purple potato flakes on antioxidant status in F344 rats fed a cholesterol-rich diet." Br J Nutr. 2007 Nov;98(5):914-21.

Harmon, K. G. et al. "Incidence of sudden cardiac death in national collegiate athletic association athletes," Circulation 123, no. 15 (April 2011): 1594–600, www.ncbi.nlm.nih.gov/pubmed/21464047.

Harris, W. S. "Fish oils and plasma lipid and lipoprotein metabolism in humans: a critical review," Journal of Lipid Research 30, no. 6 (June 1989): 785–807, http://www.ncbi.nlm.nih.gov/pubmed/2677200.

Harvie MN et al, "The effects of intermittent or continuous energy restriction on weight loss and metabolic disease risk markers: a randomized trial in young overweight women.", Int J Obes (Lond). 2011 May;35(5):714-27

Harvie MN et al, "The effect of intermittent energy and carbohydrate restriction v. daily energy restriction on weight loss and metabolic disease risk markers in overweight women.", Br J Nutr. 2013 Oct;110(8):1534-47

Haub, Carl (November/December 2002). "How Many People Have Ever Lived on Earth?" (http://www.prb.org/pdf/PT_novdec02.pdf). Population Today (Population Reference Bureau), accessed 21 January 2015

"Health benefits of taking probiotics. (n.d.)." Retrieved September 26, 2014, from http://www.health.harvard.edu/fhg/updates/update0905c.shtml

Heilbronn, L. K., and L. V. Campbell. "Adipose tissue macrophages, low grade inflammation, and insulin resistance in human obesity," Current Pharmaceutical Design 14, no. 12 (2008):1225–30, http://www.ncbi.nlm.nih.gov/pubmed/18473870.

Higdon, PhD, J. (n.d.). "Essential Fatty Acids," Linus Pauling Institute Micronutrient Research for Optimum Health. Retrieved September 20, 2014, from http://lpi.oregonstate.edu/infocenter/othernuts/omega3fa/

Holick MF, Chen TC: "Vitamin D deficiency: a worldwide problem with health consequences." Am J Clin Nutr 2008

Hoffenberg EJ, MacKenzie T, Barriga KJ, Eisenbarth GS, Bao F, Haas JE, Erlich H, Bugawan Tl T, Sokol RJ, Taki I, Norris JM, Rewers M. "A prospective study of the incidence of childhood celiac disease." J Pediatr 2003 143:308-314.

Horn, Thelma S. "Advances in Sport Psychology", Human Kinetics, 2002.

Houghton LA, Vieth R: "The case against ergocalciferol (vitamin D2) as a vitamin supplement." Am J Clin Nutr 2006

"How smoking causes cancer", Cancer Research UK Website, retrieved 10 January, 2015, from http://www.cancerresearchuk.org/about-cancer/causes-of-cancer/smoking-and-cancer/how-smoking-causes-cancer.

Hurst R, Armah CN, Dainty JR, et al; "Establishing optimal selenium status: results of a randomized, double-blind", Am J Clin Nutr. 2010 Apr;91(4):923-31. Epub 2010 Feb 24.

Inomata N. "Wheat allergy." Cur Opin Aller Clinic Immunol 2009

Institute of Medicine, Food and Nutrition Board. Dietary Reference Intakes: Calcium, Phosphorus, Magnesium, Vitamin D, and Fluoride. National Academy Press, Washington, DC, 2010.

"International tables of glycemic index and glycemic load values: 2008" by Fiona S. Atkinson, Kaye Foster-Powell, and Jennie C. Brand-Miller in the December 2008 issue of Diabetes Care, Vol. 31, number 12, pages 2281-2283

Iwane M, Arita M, Tomimoto S, Matsumoto M, Miyashita K, Nishio I. "Walking 10,000 steps/day or more reduces blood pressure and sympathetic nerve activity in mild essential hypertension.", Hypertens Res. 2000 Nov;23(6):573-80.

Jaminet, Paul and Shou-Ching Jaminet "Perfect Health Diet : Regain Health and Lose Weight by Eating the Way You Were Meant to Eat" (Scribe 2013)

Jassal DS et al., "Cardiac injury markers in nonelite marathon runners." Int J Sports Med 2009

John P Buckley, Alan Hedge, Thomas Yates, Robert J Copeland, Michael Loosemore, Mark Hamer, Gavin Bradley, David W Dunstan "The sedentary office: a growing case for change towards better health and productivity. Expert statement commissioned by Public Health England and the Active Working Community Interest Company", Br J Sports Med bjsports-2015-094618 Published Online First: 1 June 2015

Jönsson T, Granfeldt Y, Ahrén B, Branell UC, Pålsson G, Hansson A, Söderström M, Lindeberg S. "Beneficial effects of a Paleolithic diet on cardiovascular risk factors in type 2 diabetes: a randomized cross-over pilot study.", Cardiovasc Diabetol. 2009 Jul 16;8:35.

Jönsson T, Granfeldt Y, Lindeberg S, Hallberg AC. "Subjective satiety and other experiences of a Paleolithic diet compared to a diabetes diet in patients with type 2 diabetes.", Nutr J. 2013 Jul 29

Jönsson T, Granfeldt Y, Erlanson-Albertsson C, Ahrén B, Lindeberg S. "A paleolithic diet is more satiating per calorie than a mediterranean-like diet in individuals with ischemic heart disease.", Nutr Metab (Lond). 2010 Nov 30

Kallerud, Heidi and Gleeson, Nigel, "Effects of Stretching on Performances Involving Stretch-Shortening Cycles", Sports Medicine, August 2013, Volume 43, Issue 8, pp 733-750

Kanis J, Johnell O, Oden A, Jonsson B, Laet C and Dawson A, 2000. "Risk of hip fracture according to the World Health Organisation criteria for osteopenia and osteoporosis." Bone 27, pp.585-590

Katzmarzyk PT1, Church TS, Craig CL, Bouchard C. "Sitting time and mortality from all causes, cardiovascular disease, and cancer.", Med Sci Sports Exerc. 2009 May

Kessler, David A. "The End of Overeating: Taking Control of Our Insatiable Appetite." New York: Penguin, 2010.

Keukens E. A. et al. "Molecular basis of glycoalkaloid induced membrane disruption," Biochimica et Biophysica Acta 1240, no. 2 (December 1995), 216–28, http://www.ncbi.nlm.nih.gov/pubmed/8541293.

Klenke, Leslie "Paleo Girl: Take a Leap. Empower Yourself. Be Awesome!" Primal Blueprint Publishing (June 2014)

Klok, M. D. et al. "The role of leptin and ghrelin in the regulation of food intake and body weight in humans: a review," Obesity Review 8, no. 1 (January 2007): 21–34, http://www.ncbi.nlm.nih.gov/pubmed/17212793.

Klonoff DC. "The Beneficial Effects of a Paleolithic Diet on Type 2 Diabetes and Other Risk Factors for Cardiovascular Disease. Journal of Diabetes Science and Technology." 2009;3(6):1229-1232.

Knowler WC, Barrett-Connor E, Fowler SE, et al. Reduction in the incidence of type 2 diabetes with lifestyle intervention or metformin. N Engl J Med 2002; 346:393.

Kolaczynski, J. W. et al. "Acute effect of ethanol on counterregulatory response and recovery from insulin-induced hypoglycemia," Journal of Clinical Endocrinology and Metabolism 67, no. 2 (August 1988) 384–88, http://www.ncbi.nlm.nih.gov/pubmed/3292563.

Kowalski LM1, Bujko J. "Evaluation of biological and clinical potential of paleolithic diet.", Rocz Panstw Zakl Hig. 2012

Kreider RB, Serra M, Beavers KM, Moreillon J, Kresta JY, Byrd M, Oliver JM, Gutierrez J, Hudson G, Deike E, Shelmadine B, Leeke P, Rasmussen C, Greenwood M, Cooke MB, Kerksick C, Campbell JK, Beiseigel J, Jonnalagadda SS: "A structured diet and exercise program promotes favorable changes in weight loss, body composition, and weight maintenance." J Am Diet Assoc 2011

L.A. Bazzano, T. Hu, K. Reynolds, L. Yao, C. Bunol, Y. Liu, C.S. Chen, M.J. Klag, P.K. Whelton, and J. He, "Effects of Low-Carbohydrate and Low-Fat Diets. A Randomized Trial.", Ann Intern Med. 2014;161:I-22. doi:10.7326/P14-9029.

L. Maintz and N. Novak, "Histamine and histamine intolerance,"Am Jour of Clin Nutr, 2007, May; 85 (5): 1185–96.

Laitinen, K. and M Välimäki. "Bone and the 'comforts of life,'" Annals of Medicine 25, no. 4, (August 1993): 413–25, http://www.ncbi.nlm.nih.gov/pubmed/8217108.

Lehmann U, Hirche F, Stangl GI, et al: "Bioavailability of vitamin D(2) and D(3) in healthy volunteers, a randomized placebo-controlled trial." J Clin Endocrinol Metab 2013

Lewin, Alex. "Real Food Fermentation: Preserving Whole Fresh Food with Live Cultures in Your Home Kitchen", (Quarry Books July 1, 2012)

Lieberman, Daniel E. et al. "Foot strike patterns and collision forces in habitual barefoot versus shod runners," Nature 463 (January 28, 2010): 531–35, http://barefootrunning.fas.harvard.edu/Nature2010_FootStrikePatternsandCollisionF orces.pdf.

Lim SS, Vos T, Flaxman AD, Danaei G, Shibuya K, Adair-Rohani H et al. "A comparative risk assessment of burden of disease and injury attributable to 67 risk factors and risk factor clusters in 21 regions, 1990-2010: a systematic analysis for the Global Burden of Disease Study 2010." Lancet, 2012

Lindeberg, S "The Kitava Study" http://www.staffanlindeberg.com/TheKitavaStudy.html

Lindeberg, S, Jönsson, T, Granfeldt, Y, Borgstrand, E, Soffman, J, Sjöström, K, and Ahrén, B. "A Palaeolithic diet improves glucose tolerance more than a Mediterranean-like diet in individuals with ischaemic heart disease." Diabetologia, 2007

Lindeberg, S, Cordain, L, and Eaton, SB. "Biological and clinical potential of a palaeolithic diet." J Nutr Environ Med, 2003;

Lionel Bey andMarc T. Hamilton. "Suppression of skeletal muscle lipoprotein lipase activity during physical inactivity: a molecular reason to maintain daily low-intensity activity.", J Physiol (2003), 551.2, pp. 673–682

Liu S, Willett WC. "Dietary glycemic load and atherothrombotic risk." Curr Atheroscler Rep. 2002

Logan VF, Gray AR, Peddie MC, et al: "Long-term vitamin D3 supplementation is more effective than vitamin D2 in maintaining serum 25-hydroxyvitamin D status over the winter months." Br J Nutr 2013

Ludvigsson et al, 2012. "The Oslo definitions for coeliac disease and related terms.", Gut doi:10.1136/gutjnl-2011-301346

Ludwig DS. "The glycemic index: physiological mechanisms relating to obesity, diabetes, and cardiovascular disease." JAMA. 2002

Ludwig DS. "Dietary glycemic index and the regulation of body weight." Lipids. 2003

Macri, Irena : "Eat Drink Paleo : Over 100 Paleo-Inspired Recipes For Everyone" (Penguin, 2015)

Majumder, K. and J. Wu. "Angiotensin I converting enzyme inhibitory peptides from simulated in vitro gastrointestinal digestion of cooked eggs," Journal of Agricultural and Food Chemistry 57, no. 2 (January 2009), 471–77, http://www.ncbi.nlm.nih.gov/pubmed/19154160.

Marcin Barański, Dominika Średnicka-Tober, Nikolaos Volakakis, Chris Seal, Roy Sanderson, Gavin B. Stewart, Charles Benbrook, Bruno Biavati, Emilia Markellou, Charilaos Giotis, Joanna Gromadzka-Ostrowska, Ewa Rembiałkowska, Krystyna Skwarło-Sońta, Raija Tahvonen, Dagmar Janovská, Urs Niggli, Philippe Nicot and Carlo Leifert, "Higher antioxidant and lower cadmium concentrations and lower incidence of pesticide residues in organically grown crops: a systematic literature review and meta-analyses.", http://dx.doi.org/10.1017/S0007114514001366, Published online: 26 June 2014

Masharani U, Sherchan P, Schloetter M, Stratford S, Xiao A, Sebastian A, Nolte Kennedy M, Frassetto L. "Metabolic and physiologic effects from consuming a hunter-gatherer (Paleolithic)-type diet in type 2 diabetes.", Eur J Clin Nutr. 2015 Apr 1

McCaw, Steven T. and Jeffery J. Friday. "A comparison of muscle activity between a free weight and machine bench press," Journal of Strength and Conditioning Research 8, no. 4 (November 1994): 259–64.

McCusker, Rachel R. Bruce A. Goldberger and Edward J. Cone. "Caffeine content of energy drinks, carbonated sodas and other beverages," Journal of Analytical Toxicology 30, no. 2. (March 2006): 112–14, http://jat.oxfordjournals.org/content/30/2/112.full.pdf+html.

Mellberg C, Sandberg S, Ryberg M, Eriksson M, Brage S, Larsson C, Olsson T, Lindahl B. "Long-term effects of a Palaeolithic-type diet in obese postmenopausal women: a 2-year randomized trial.", Eur J Clin Nutr. 2014 Mar

Middleton N et al., "Altered left ventricular diastolic filling following a marathon is a reproducible phenomenon." Int J Cardiol. 2007 Oct 31;122(1):87-9. Epub 2007 Jan 11.

Millar L, Kremer P, de Silva-Sanigorski A, McCabe MP, Mavoa H, Moodie M, Utter J, Bell C, Malakellis M, Mathews L, Roberts G, Robertson N, Swinburn BA. "Reduction in overweight and obesity from a 3-year community-based intervention in Australia: The 'It's Your Move!' project." Obes Rev 2011

Mills EJ, Rachlis B, Wu P, Devereaux PJ, Arora P, Perri D. "Primary prevention of cardiovascular mortality and events with statin treatments: a network meta-analysis involving more than 65,000 patients." J Am Coll Cardiol. 2008 Nov 25;52(22):1769-81. PubMed PMID: 19022156.

Mittlestaedt, Martin. "Canada first to declare bisphenol A toxic," Globe and Mail, August, 2010, http://www.theglobeandmail.com/technology/science/canada-first-to-declare-bisphenol-a-toxic/article1214889.

Mitka M. "Some question use of statins to reduce cardiovascular risks in healthy women." JAMA. 2012 Mar 7;307(9):893-4

"Mediterranean Diet vs. Paleolithic Diet vs. Standard American Diet. (n.d.)." Retrieved October 7, 2014, from http://thepaleodiet.com/mediterranean-diet-vs-paleolithic-diet-vs-standard-american-diet/.

Mora-Ripoll R, "The therapeutic value of laughter in medicine.", Altern Ther Health Med. 2010 Nov-Dec;16(6):56-64.

Mozaffarian D, Fahimi S, Singh GM, Micha R, Khatibzadeh S, Engell RE, Lim S, et al.; "Global Burden of Diseases Nutrition and Chronic Diseases Expert Group. Global sodium consumption and death from cardiovascular causes." N Engl J Med. 2014;371(7):624–34

Moore, E. "Leaky gut syndrome: using probiotics and digestive enzymes in autoimmune disorders," General Medicine (2007).

Moore, Jimmy Westman, Eric "Cholesterol Clarity: What the HDL is Wrong with My Numbers?", (Victory Belt Publishing 2013).

Moore, Jimmy Westman, Eric "Keto Clarity: Your Definitive Guide to the Benefits of a low-carb, high-fat diet", (Victory Belt Publishing 2014).

Nakano, Y. et al. "A functional variant in the human betacellulin gene promoter is associated with type 2 diabetes," Diabetes 54, no. 12 (December 2005): 3560–66, http://www.ncbi.nlm.nih.gov/pubmed/16306376.

"National Center for Health Statistics, National Office of Vital Statistics," Published 1947, available from http://www.cdc.gov/nchs/data/statab/lead1900_98.pdf.

National Hip Fracture Database, "National Hip Fracture Database (NHFD) extended report 2014.", London: Royal College of Physicians.

National Osteoporosis Foundation, "Break Free from Osteoporosis." Accessed May 2014, http://nof.org/connect.

National Osteoporosis Society "Annual Review 2013," available at: http://www.nos.org.uk/document.doc?id=1625

NCD Alliance, "The Global Epidemic," accessed April 2014, http://www.ncdalliance.org/globalepidemic.

Noakes, Creed, Proudfoot "The Real Meal Revolution: The Radical, Sustainable Approach to Healthy Eating" (Robinson, 2015)

O. De Schutter and G. Vanloqueren, "The New Green Revolution: How twenty-first-century science can feed the world", Resilience, Aug 21, 2011. Retrieved Sept 17, 2014, from http://www.resilience.org/stories/2011-08-21/new-green-revolution-how-twenty-first-century-science-can-geed-world.

"Obesity and Overweight" fact sheet, World Health Organization, published May 2012, http://www.who.int/mediacentre/factsheets/fs311/en.

"Obesity and the Economics of Prevention: Fit Not Fat," Organisation for Economic Co-operation and Development, published September 23, 2010, http://www.oecd.org/health/healthpoliciesanddata/obesityandtheeconomicsofpreventionfitnotfat.htm.

Oda, K. et al. "Adjuvant and haemolytic activities of 47 saponins derived from medicinal and food plants," Biological Chemistry 381, no. 1 (January 2000): 67–74, http://www.ncbi.nlm.nih.gov/pubmed/10722052.

Office of National Statistics, 2014. Annual Mid-year Population Estimates, 2013. Accessed November 2014, http://www.ons.gov.uk/ons/rel/pop-estimate/population-estimates-for-uk--england-and-wales--scotland-and-northern-ireland/2013/stb---mid-2013-uk-population-estimates.html

O'Keefe JH et al., "Achieving hunter-gatherer fitness in the 21st century: back to the future." Am J Med 2010.

O'Keefe, S. J., and V. Marks. "Lunchtime gin and tonic a cause of reactive hypoglycemia," Lancet 1 no. 8025 (June 1977), 1286–88, http://www.ncbi.nlm.nih.gov/pubmed/68385.

Okada, H., Kuhn, C., Feillet, H., & Bach, J. (2010, January 21). "The 'hygiene hypothesis' for auto-immune and related disease: An update." Retrieved September 25, 2014, from http://www.ncbi.nlm.nih.gov/pmc/articles/PMC2841828/.

Okuyama, H. et al. "Dietary fatty acids—the N-6/N-3 balance and chronic elderly diseases. Excess linoleic acid and relative N-3 deficiency syndrome seen in Japan," Progress in Lipid Research 35, no. 4 (December 1996): 409–57, http://www.ncbi.nlm.nih.gov/pubmed/9246358.

Österdahl, M. et al. "Effects of a short-term intervention with a Paleolithic diet in healthy volunteers," European Journal of Clinical Nutrition 62, no. 5 (May 2008): 682–85, http://www.ncbi.nlm.nih.gov/pubmed/17522610.

P. Gadsby and L. Steele, "The Inuit Paradox", *Discover Magazine* (Oct 1, 2004). Retrieved October 7, 2014, from http://discovermagazine.com/2004/oct/inuit-paradox.

Paleo Foundation, paleocertified.com and certifiedpaleo.com, accessed January 2015

Pastore RL, et al. Nutr Res. 2015, "Paleolithic nutrition improves plasma lipid concentrations of hypercholesterolemic adults to a greater extent than traditional heart-healthy dietary recommendations." Nutr Res. 2015 May 14

Patel, B. "Potato glycoalkaloids adversely affect intestinal permeability and aggravate inflammatory bowel disease," Inflammatory Bowel Diseases 8, no. 5 (September 2002), 340–46, http://www.ncbi.nlm.nih.gov/pubmed/12479649.

Perrier, E. T. et al. "The acute effects of a warm-up including static or dynamic stretching on countermovement jump height, reaction time, and flexibility," Journal of Strength and Conditioning Research 25, no. 5 (July 2011): 1925–31, http://www.ncbi.nlm.nih.gov/pubmed/21701282.

Perlmutter, David "Grain Brain : The Surprising Truth about Wheat, Carbs, and Sugar - Your Brain's Silent Killers", (Yellow Kite, Jan 2014)

"Physical Activity Guidelines Advisory Committee. Physical Activity Guidelines Advisory Committee Report", 2008. Washington, DC: U.S. Department of Health and Human Services;2008. Available from: http://www.health.gov/paguidelines/Report/pdf/CommitteeReport.pdf

Pleasance, E. D. et al. "A small-cell lung cancer genome with complex signatures of tobacco exposure," Nature 423, no. 7278 (January 2010): 184–90, http://www.ncbi.nlm.nih.gov/pubmed/20016488.

"Population Reference Bureau" (http://www.prb.org/Articles/2002/HowManyPeopleHaveEverLivedonEarth.aspx). Prb.org.2002-12-01, accessed 21 January 2015

Price, Weston. "Nutrition and Physical Degeneration: A Comparison of Primitive and Modern Diets and Their Effects." 8th ed. Price Pottenger Nutrition Foundation, 2008.

"Public Awareness of Clinical Research," (2005) Retrieved 15 February 2015, from http://www.ukcrc.org/patients-and-public/public-awareness-of-clinical-research/.

Q. Yang, Z. Zhang, E. W. Gregg, W. D. Flanders, R. Merritt, F. B. Hu, "Added sugar intake and cardiovascular diseases mortality among adults," JAMA Intern Med, 2014; 174 (4): 516–524.

Ratel, S. et al. "High-intensity intermittent activities at school: controversies and facts," Journal of Sports Medicine and Physical Fitness 44, no. 3 (September 2004), 272–80, http://www.ncbi.nlm.nih.gov/pubmed/15756166.

Ray KK, Seshasai SR, Erqou S, Sever P, Jukema JW, Ford I, Sattar N. Statins and all-cause mortality in high-risk primary prevention: a meta-analysis of 11 randomized controlled trials involving 65,229 participants. Arch Intern Med. 2010 Jun 28;170(12):1024-31. Review. PubMed PMID: 20585067.

Redberg RF, Katz MH. "Healthy men should not take statins." JAMA. 2012;307(14):1491-2

Richards, Byron, and Mary Richards. "Mastering Leptin: Your Guide to Permanent Weight Loss and Optimum Health." 3rd ed. Minneapolis, MN: Wellness Resources, 2009.

Richards, C. E. et al. "Is your prescription of distance running shoes evidence based?" British Journal of Sports Medicine 43, no. 3 (March 2009): 159–62, http://www.ncbi.nlm.nih.gov/pubmed/18424485.

Ridker et al. "Rosuvastatin to prevent vascular events in men and women with elevated c-reactive protein." NEJM. 2008; 359(21): 2195-2207.

Rivas DA, Fielding RA. "Exercise as a countermeasure for sarcopenia. In: Lynch GS, ed. Sarcopenia — Age-Related Muscle Wasting and Weakness." New York, NY; Springer; 2011:333-372.

Robbins, S. et al. "Athletic footwear affects balance in men," British Journal of Sports Medicine 28, no. 2 (June 1994): 117–22, http://www.ncbi.nlm.nih.gov/pmc/articles/PMC1332044/.

Room, R. et al. "Alcohol and public health," Lancet 365, no. 9458 (February 2005): 519–30, doi:10.1016/S0140-6736(08)61345-8.

Rudelle, S. et al. "Effect of a thermogenic beverage on 24-hour energy metabolism in humans," Obesity (Silver Spring) 15, no. 2 (February 2007): 349–55, http://www.ncbi.nlm.nih.gov/pubmed/17299107.

Ryan-Harshman M, Aldoori W; "The relevance of selenium to immunity, cancer, and infectious/inflammatory diseases." Can J Diet Pract Res. 2005 Summer;66(2):98-102.

Sale, D., and D. MacDougall. (1981). "Specificity in strength training: a review for the coach and athlete," Canadian Journal of Applied Sport Sciences 6 (June 1981): 87–92.

Sanfilippo, Diane "Practical Paleo : A Practical Approach to Health and a Whole-Foods Lifestyle" (Victory Belt Publishing 2012)

Sapone et al., "Spectrum of gluten-related disorders: consensus on new nomenclature and classification.", BMC Medicine 2012, 10:13, http://www.biomedcentral.com/1741-7015/10/13

Sarah N Stabler, Aaron M Tejani, Fong Huynh and Claire Fowkes, "Garlic for the prevention of cardiovascular morbidity and mortality in hypertensive patients." Retrieved 11 November, 2014, from http://onlinelibrary.wiley.com/doi/10.1002/14651858.CD007653.pub2/full.

Sartori, S. B., Whittle, N., Hetzenauer, A., & Singewald, N. (2012). Magnesium deficiency induces anxiety and HPA axis dysregulation: Modulation by therapeutic drug treatment. Neuropharmacology, 62(1), 304–312. doi:10.1016/j.neuropharm.2011.07.027

Sarubin Fragaakis A, Thomson C. The Health Professional's Guide to Popular Dietary Supplements. 3rd ed. Chicago, IL: American Dietetic Association; 2007.

Satoh, N. et al. "Sympathetic activation of leptin via the ventromedial hypothalamus: leptin-induced increase in catecholamine secretion," Diabetes 48, no. 9 (September 1999): 1787–93, http://www.ncbi.nlm.nih.gov/pubmed/10480609.

Schlosser, Eric. Fast Food Nation: "What The All-American Meal Is Doing to the World." London: Penguin, 2002.

Schmid D et al., "Television Viewing and Time Spent Sedentary in Relation to Cancer Risk: A Meta-Analysis", JNCI J Natl Cancer Inst (2014).

Schmidt, Richard A. and Timothy D. Lee. "Motor Control and Learning: A Behavioral Emphasis," 5th ed. Champaign, IL: Human Kinetics, March 30, 2011.

Schmulson, M. J. "Brain-gut interaction in irritable bowel syndrome: new findings of a multicomponent disease model," Israel Medical Association Journal 3, no. 2 (February 2001): 104–10, http://www.ncbi.nlm.nih.gov/pubmed/11347592.

Schwarz, Barry. "The Paradox of Choice: Why More is Less." New York: HarperCollins, 2005.

"Second National Report on Biochemical Indicators of Diet and Nutrition in the U.S. Population 2012." Available from: http://www.cdc.gov/nutritionreport/pdf/Nutrition_Book_complete508_final.pdf

Sherwood, Lauralee. "Fundamentals of Physiology: A Human Perspective." 3rd ed. Independence, KY: Cengage Learning, 2006.

Shin JY, Xun P, Nakamura Y, He K. "Egg consumption in relation to risk of cardiovascular disease and diabetes: a systematic review and meta-analysis." Am J Clin Nutr. 2013;98(1):146-59. PMID: 23676423.

Shiraev, T et al., "Evidence Based Exercise: Clinical Benefits of High Intensity Interval Training", AFP 41, (December 2012)

Shoba G1, Joy D, Joseph T, Majeed M, Rajendran R, Srinivas PS. "Influence of piperine on the pharmacokinetics of curcumin in animals and human volunteers.", Planta Med. 1998 May;64(4):353-6.

Sieri S, Krogh V, Berrino F, et al. "Dietary glycemic load and index and risk of coronary heart disease in a large Italian cohort: the EPICOR study." Arch Intern Med. 2010

Siler, S. Q. et al. "De novo lipogenesis, lipid kinetics, and whole-body lipid balances in humans after acute alcohol consumption," American Journal of Clinical Nutrition 70, no. 5 (November 1999): 928–36, http://www.ncbi.nlm.nih.gov/pubmed/10539756.

Simopoulos, AP, et al. "The importance of the omega-3/omega-6 fatty acid ratio in cardiovascular disease and other chronic diseases," Experimental Biology and Medicine 233, no. 6 (June 2008): 674–88, http://www.ncbi.nlm.nih.gov/pubmed/18408140.

Sisson, Mark. "The Primal Blueprint: Reprogram your genes for effortless weight loss, vibrant health, and boundless energy." Primal Nutrition, Inc, 2012.

Smith, David A. "Folic acid fortification: the good, the bad, and the puzzle of vitamin B-12", Am J Clin Nutr January 2007 vol. 85 (1) 3-5.

Spiegel K, Tasali E, Penev P "Sleep curtailment in healthy young men is associated with decreased leptin levels, elevated ghrelin levels and increased hunger and appetite." Annals of internal Medicine. Dec 2004 Vol. 141 (11) -846 – 851

Srinivasan K "Black pepper and its pungent principle-piperine: a review of diverse physiological effects.", Crit Rev Food Sci Nutr. 2007;47(8):735-48.

Stipp, David. "How Intermittent Fasting Might Help You Live a Longer and Healthier Life", http://www.scientificamerican.com/article/how-intermittent-fasting-might-help-you-live-longer-healthier-life/. Published online Dec 18, 2012.

Sun MX, Huang XQ, Yan Y, Li BW, Zhong WJ, Chen JF, Zhang YM, Wang ZZ, Wang L, Shi XC, Li J, Xie MH. "One-hour after-school exercise ameliorates central adiposity and lipids in overweight Chinese adolescents: a randomized controlled trial." Chin Med J 2011

Susan G. Lakoski, Benjamin L. Willis, Carolyn E. Barlow, David Leonard, Ang Gao, Nina B. Radford, Stephen W. Farrell, Pamela S. Douglas, Jarett D. Berry, Laura F. DeFina, Lee W. Jones, "Midlife Cardiorespiratory Fitness, Incident Cancer, and Survival After Cancer in Men", JAMA Oncol. Published online March 26, 2015. doi:10.1001/jamaoncol.2015.0226

"Sweet Potato or Yam? Which is which?". Foodreference.com. 20 March 2007. Retrieved 12 September 2014.

Tabata, I. et al. "Effects of moderate-intensity endurance and high-intensity intermittent training on anaerobic capacity and VO2max," Medicine and Science in Sports and Exercise 28, no. 10 (October 1996): 1327–30, http://www.ncbi.nlm.nih.gov/pubmed/8897392.

Taheri, S. "Short sleep duration is associated with reduced leptin, elevated ghrelin, and increased body mass index," PLOS Medicine 1, no. 3 (December 2004): e62, http://www.ncbi.nlm.nih.gov/pubmed/15602591.

Tanabe S. "Analysis of food allergen structures and development of foods for allergic patients." Biosci Biotechnol Biochem 2008

Tatham AS, Shewry PR. "Allergens in wheat and related cereals." Clin Experiment Aller 2008, 38

Taylor F, Ward K, Moore TH, Burke M, Davey Smith G, Casas JP, Ebrahim S. "Statins for the primary prevention of cardiovascular disease." Cochrane Database Syst Rev. 2011 Jan 19;(1):CD004816. Review. PubMed PMID: 21249663.

Teede H, Deeks A, Moran L, "Polycystic ovary syndrome: a complex condition with psychological, reproductive and metabolic manifestations that impacts on health across the lifespan" (2010) BMC Med 8 (1): 41.

Temme, E. H., and P. G. Van Hoydonck. "Tea consumption and iron status," European Journal of Clinical Nutrition 56, no. 5 (May 2002): 379–86, http://www.ncbi.nlm.nih.gov/pubmed/12001007.

Thavendiranathan P. "Primary prevention of cardiovascular disease with statin therapy". Arch Int Med. 2006; 166: 2307-13.

"The Impact of Chronic Disease in the United Kingdom" from http://www.who.int/chp/chronic_disease_report/media/uk.pdf (Accessed April 2015)

Thompson Coon, J. et al. "Does participating in physical activity in outdoor natural environments have a greater effect on physical and mental wellbeing than physical activity indoors? A systematic review," Environmental Science & Technology 45, no. 5 (March 2011): 1761–72, www.ncbi.nlm.nih.gov/pubmed/21291246.

Trapp, E. G. et al. "The effects of high-intensity intermittent exercise training on fat loss and fasting insulin levels of young women." International Journal of Obesity 32, no. 4 (April 2008): 684–91

Tripkovic L, Lambert H, Hart K, et al: "Comparison of vitamin D2 and vitamin D3 supplementation in raising serum 25-hydroxyvitamin D status: a systematic review and meta-analysis." Am J Clin Nutr 2012

"Update on Bisphenol A for Use in Food Contact Applications," U.S. Food and Drug Administration website, January 2010, last modified April 2, 2012, http://www.fda.gov/newsevents/publichealthfocus/ucm064437.htm.

USDA National Nutrient Database for Standard Reference, last modified December 2011, http://ndb.nal.usda.gov. (Multiple Access).

"USDA Scientific Report of the 2015 Dietary Guidelines Advisory Committee", available from http://www.health.gov/dietaryguidelines/2015-scientific-report/PDFs/Scientific-Report-of-the-2015-Dietary-Guidelines-Advisory-Committee.pdf (Multiple Access).

U. Ravnskov et al., "The statin-low cholesterol-cancer conundrum", Monthly Journal of the Association of Physicians, December 2011, 8 March 2015, http://qjmed.oxfordjournals.org/content/qjmed/early/2011/12/08/qjmed.hcr243.ful l.pdf.

Vaarala, O. et al. "Cow's milk formula feeding induces primary immunization to insulin in infants at genetic risk for type 1 diabetes," Diabetes 48, no. 7 (July 1999): 1389–94, http://www.ncbi.nlm.nih.gov/pubmed/10389843.

Vedhara, K et al. "Personality and gene expression: Do individual differences exist in the leukocyte transcriptome?", Psychoneuroendocrinology. 2015 Feb

Virtanen, S. M. et al. "Early introduction of dairy products associated with increased risk of IDDM in Finnish children," Diabetes 42, no. 12 (December 1993): 1786–90, http://www.ncbi.nlm.nih.gov/pubmed/8243824.

Vlachopoulos C, Xaplanteris P, Alexopoulos N, Aznaouridis K, Vasiliadou C, Baou K, Stefanadi E, Stefanadis C. "Divergent effects of laughter and mental stress on arterial stiffness and central hemodynamics.", Psychosom Med. 2009 May;71(4):446-53.

"Yams Nutrition Facts", http://www.nutrition-and-you.com/yams.html. Retrieved 12 September 2014.

Yang Q, Zhang Z, Gregg EW, Flanders W, Merritt R, Hu FB. "Added Sugar Intake and Cardiovascular Diseases Mortality Among US Adults." JAMA Intern Med. 2014;174(4):516-524. doi:10.1001/jamainternmed.2013.13563. Retrieved September 28, 2014.

Wahls, Terry "The Wahls Protocol: A Radical New Way to Treat All Chronic Autoimmune Conditions Using Paleo Principles" (Avery, 2015)

Wal JM "Bovine milk allergenicity". Ann. Allergy Asthma Immunol. 93 (5 Suppl 3): S2–11 (Nov 2004)

Wansink, Brian. "Mindless Eating: Why We Eat More Than We Think." New York: Bantam, 2006.

"We Love Paleo", International Film Documentary, http://bit.ly/WeLovePaleo

"What is Adrenal Fatigue?" Retrieved September 17, 2014, from http://www.adrenalfatigue.org/what-is-adrenal-fatigue.

Wilson, Edward O. "Biophilia: The Human Bond With Other Species" (Harvard University Press, January 1984).

"WHO calls on countries to reduce sugars intake among adults and children," (March 2015) from http://www.who.int/mediacentre/news/releases/2015/sugar-guideline/en/. (Accessed 2 April, 2015).

Wolf, Robb. "The Paleo Solution: The Original Human Diet." Las Vegas: Victory Belt, 2010.

Zarich, S. W. "Metabolic syndrome, diabetes, and cardiovascular events: current controversies, and recommendations," Minerva Cardioangiologica 54, no. 2 (April 2006): 195–214, http://www.ncbi.nlm.nih.gov/pubmed/16778752.

Zderic W Theodore, Hamilton T Marc. "Identification of hemostatic genes expressed in human and rat leg muscles and a novel gene (LPP1/PAP2A) suppressed during prolonged physical inactivity (sitting)." Lipids in Health and Disease 2012, 11:137

ABOUT THE AUTHOR

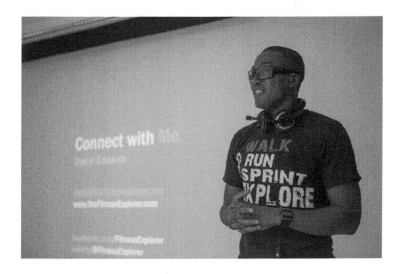

Darryl Edwards, owner of *Fitness Explorer Training & Nutrition*, founder of *HEALTH Unplugged* and creator of *Primal Play*. Darryl is an international speaker, certified personal trainer, nutritional therapist, and best-selling author of *Paleo Fitness : Primal Training And Nutrition To Get Lean, Strong And Healthy*. *Paleo Fitness* was awarded Best Fitness Book and Darryl was

nominated as Health Hero of the Year at the ***Paleo f(x)***
2015 awards show. Darryl's work has been published in
titles such as *Men's Fitness*, *Women's Health*, *Elle*, *Top Santé*,
Experience Life, featured on the BBC radio and TV in the
UK, and ABC in Australia. He also appears in the 2015
international documentary film *We Love Paleo* and serves
on the Primal Blueprint Expert Certification advisory
board.

Over ten years ago Darryl embarked on a Paleo
approach to well-being when he had no choice but to
focus on his health. Back then he was diagnosed with
iron-deficiency anaemia, lived with hypertension, had an
elevated cardiovascular disease risk profile and 26 per
cent body fat, most of it around the middle. He felt weak
and lethargic, and suffered from insomnia. He endured
low back pain and would often encounter excruciating
knee pain when taking part in most activities. He even
began to wear knee supports to walk short distances and
to walk up stairs.

It didn't take long after focussing on a Paleo lifestyle
to reap the benefits and improved health continues to the

present day. His body fat now averages 10 per cent, the spare tyre has disappeared, his blood pressure is now in the optimal range, and he is no longer iron-deficient anaemic. His resting heart rate is an *athletic* 38 beats per minute. He's stronger, fitter and healthier now in his forties than at any other period of his life. No more back or knee pain, increased energy levels, and a renewed sense of vitality. Other biomarkers of health such as cholesterol, blood triglycerides, fasting glucose, vitamin and mineral levels and many other parameters are within normal or optimal ranges, which had not been the case before.

He now advises people on achieving and maintaining a healthy lifestyle amidst the epidemic of obesity and other chronic lifestyle diseases and is a leading expert in the optimisation of health and wellbeing, offering one-to-one and group-based consultations.

Darryl can be found at his blog, **The Fitness Explorer** (*www.thefitnessexplorer.com*), where he documents his experience with a Paleo lifestyle. He lives in London, England.

OTHER BOOKS BY DARRYL EDWARDS

Paleo Fitness: A Primal Training and Nutrition Program to Get Lean, Strong and Healthy (Ulysses Press 2013)

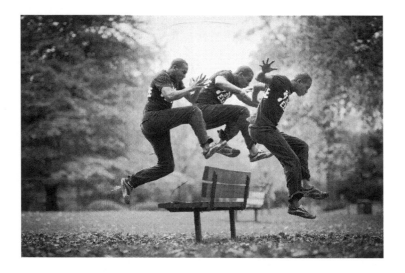